The Anti-Inflammatory Diet Cookbook for Beginners

The Anti-Inflammatory Diet Cookbook for Beginners

Natural Treatments for Chronic Inflammation, 100 Easy and Delicious Recipes That Reduce Inflammation

Tina Cooper

Table of Contents

Introduction

If you take a moment to browse the web and check out some health-related statistics, you would immediately notice that more than 44 million people in the US alone suffer from Arthritis while another 25 million suffer from Asthma. The numbers go much higher if you take the global population into account.

What most people don't understand, though, is that most of these diseases are very closely linked to a very serious issue that they tend to ignore, chronic inflammation.

Even though people are aware of it, most of the time, they seem to just ignore the effects of inflammation until it's too late.

However, as more and more research is conducted, people are becoming more aware of the situation and harmful side effects that entail chronic inflammation and are slowly taking steps to reduce it.

With that in mind, an individuals' mindset is slowly changing. Americans are looking for newer and more efficient ways to alter their unhealthy lifestyles and decrease their chances of suffering from inflammation.

While many factors come into play here, what you eat and how you eat plays a key role in maintaining a healthy body.

The Anti-Inflammatory diet understands this perfectly and is designed to encourage you to adopt a new, healthier lifestyle and dietary plan that will allow your body to develop resistance against chronic inflammation.

This book has been designed to act as a one-stop entry point into the world of the Anti-Inflammatory diet; therefore, I have covered all the basic concepts and fundamentals of inflammation and the diet in the first introductory chapters. This information should give you a good idea of what inflammation is, why it is harmful, and how this diet can help you tackle it.

Once you are done with the introductory chapters, you will find a fine collection of Anti-Inflammatory recipes that will inspire you to have a healthy journey without sacrificing any flavor from your life!

Thanks to the large variety of recipes, you are sure to find something that you will love. Thank you for your support, and I sincerely hope that you enjoy this book!

Chapter 1: Preparing for the Anti-Inflammatory Diet

What is the Anti-Inflammatory Diet?

Unlike most of the diets out there that follow an extremely tight dietary routine, the Anti-Inflammatory diet is pretty simple and straight forward.

The main goal of the Anti-Inflammatory Diet program is to basically show you the foods that you should consume to stay healthy. More specifically, the program essentially encourages you to consume foods that will lower the possibility of an uncontrolled inflammatory response.

A properly prepared and well-balanced Anti-Inflammatory Diet is rich in food that is packed with anti-oxidants.

These anti-oxidants are basically reactive molecules present in food that help your body reduce the number of cell-damaging free radicals present in your body.

The Sudden Interest in Anti-Inflammatory Diet

So, why are people looking for an Anti-Inflammatory diet? Well, it's pretty clear, really!

Despite having the best technology and health care services globally, America is still suffering from an Epidemic of Chronic Inflammation and other Chronic Inflammatory diseases.

The change in the form of our citizens' modern diet is greatly contributing to increasing the number of incidents as well.

And when we talk about Chronic Inflammation, we're talking about many different diseases, such as arthritis, asthma, etc.

In the US alone, nearly 43 million people suffer from arthritis, and 25 million suffer from asthma.

Those are no small numbers, and the Americans' need to find a proper solution for the Anti-Inflammatory regime is at an all-time high!

And that is exactly why the concept of the Anti-Inflammatory diet is gaining so much popularity.

Natural Treatments for Chronic Inflammation

Apart from following the amazing Anti-Inflammatory diet, there are certain other natural remedies that you might want to know, which might help you in the long run.

Now, several doctors try to recommend various anti-inflammatory drugs, such as ibuprofen, to manage and keep the pain under control. Still, these medicines don't deal with the root of the problem.

You may consider them temporary solutions, but they will essentially do more harm to your body than good in the long run.

That being said, there are some ingredients and natural remedies that you should know about, which work just as well or even better than prescribed NSAIDS!

You may use the following mentioned herbs independently, but combining them would amplify the healing properties.

Boswellia

This herb is also known as Indian Frankincense and is native to India. The herb is mostly extracted from the "Boswellia Serrata Tree."

Traditional ayurvedic scriptures hold Boswellia with very high regard for dealing with different conditions that may arise due to chronic inflammation, such as bronchitis, fever, etc.

As you can already tell, this herb is an excellent anti-inflammatory medicine and a pain reliever.

Research has shown that Boswellia Resin contains several different acids that contribute to its anti-inflammatory properties.

All around the world, Boswellia has been seen to cure ailments related to different inflammatory diseases, such as ulcerative colitis that particularly affect the digestive system.

This herb also helps improve another anti-inflammatory condition known as osteoarthritis, causing pain in the knee joint by wearing down the cartilage.

Stephania Root

This one might sound a little unique or new, but that's because this plant, "Stephania Tetrandra," is a plant that is native to the lands of Taiwan and China. But just to let you know, this is one of the most fundamental herbs used in traditional Chinese apothecary.

This herb is often used to deal with various symptoms, such as edema, asthma, headaches, indigestion, etc.

Like the others, recent studies have also shown that this root is an awesome anti-inflammatory herb. This particular herb helps reduce the production of cytokines, which I discussed earlier, which significantly increases the dire symptoms of chronic inflammation.

Other research has shown that Tetrandrine, also present in Stephania, might help with cancer by lowering the number of cells and clearing out the damaged cells.

Ginger

Ginger is already very well-known for its amazing health properties. If you have a sore throat and drink just a cup of ginger-lemon tea, you will immediately start feeling the positive effects.

Ginger is a very powerful anti-inflammatory thanks to the presence of a compound known as gingerol.

Various studies have shown that gingerol helps to deactivate a pathway known as "NF-kb" that is closely linked to inflammation caused by several different diseases, such as Alzheimer's and Diabetes.

Ginger is also seen to help reduce muscle aches after extreme workouts. Recent studies have shown that individuals who take about 2 gm of ginger every day experienced a significant decrease in muscle pain after just 11 days.

Curcumin

There is a misconception amongst people who often think that turmeric and cumin are the same ingredients, but the truth is far from it.

Curcumin, or "Cumin" as we like to call it, is an excellent anti-inflammatory and bioactive compound present in turmeric. This is the particular compound that gives the various plants their healing ability.

Chinese and Ayurvedic medicine have been utilizing turmeric for a long time, going back almost 4000 years!

These days, turmeric is used to deal with various diseases, such as urinary infection, asthma, rthritis, skin cancer, and chronic inflammation.

Curcumin is often believed to be one of the most effective and safe natural anti-inflammatories out there.

Studies show that it essentially works by restricting the creation of inflammatory proteins and cells. That being said, some of the problems that it helps to deal with include:

- Cancer
- Pancreatitis
- IBS
- Post-Surgery Inflammation
- Arthritis

Apart from all the things mentioned above, Curcumin is also an awesome natural painkiller that helps reduce pain even more effectively than ibuprofen.

Who Can it help?

While anyone can follow the Anti-Inflammatory diet just to stay healthy, you should understand that Iinflammation is caused by several different diseases, which altogether lead to the symptoms of chronic inflammation turning into something serious. So, it's rather difficult to pinpoint just several symptoms that might lead to inflammation.

However, research has shown that the following signs and symptoms are constant in individuals who suffer from chronic inflammation in the long run.

- Long-term fatigue
- Serious aches in muscles
- Continuous low-grade fever
- Redness and swelling in various regions
- Prolonged numbness in feet and hands
- Loss of hair
- The sudden appearance of skin rashes

Keep in mind that these are not the only symptoms. As I mentioned earlier, these symptoms are generally accompanied by the core symptoms of a certain disease. For example, suppose you are affected by diabetes. In that case, you might experience the symptoms mentioned above alongside the symptoms of diabetes, such as extreme weight loss, thirst, and so on.

If you happen to show any of the symptoms mentioned above, you might want to consider following the program.

Understanding the Food List

As you can already tell, the food list is at the heart of this particular diet, so you need to understand which foods are allowed and which are not.

You should be happy to know, though, that despite there being some manner of restrictions when it comes to certain food groups, you will still have the option to enjoy a great number of absolutely delicious meals to help you rejuvenate your body.

To keep things simple and easy for you to understand, let me break down the food list into separate food groups and let you know what foods you should go for and avoid.

Beans and Legumes

What to eat

- Black-eyed peas
- Red beans
- Pinto beans
- Lentils
- Chickpeas
- Black beans

What not to eat

- Nothing, in particular, to be aware of.

Fruits

What to eat

- Blueberries
- Blackberries
- Raspberries
- Strawberries
- Dark red grapes
- Cherries
- Coconut
- Avocado
- Citrus fruits

What not to eat

- Nothing, in particular, to be aware of.

Allium Vegetables

What to eat

- Onion
- Garlic
- Chives
- Shallots
- Leeks
- Green onions

What not to eat

- Nothing, in particular, to be aware of.

Vegetables

What to eat

- Cauliflower
- Broccoli
- Cabbage
- Dark leafy greens
- Mustard greens
- Collard greens
- Lettuce
- Spinach
- Mushrooms
- Squash

What not to eat

- Nothing, in particular, to be aware of.

Nightshade Vegetables

What to eat

- Tomatoes
- Bell pepper
- Eggplant
- potatoes

What not to eat

- Nothing, in particular, to be aware of. However, some individuals are a bit sensitive to certain Nightshade vegetables, so make sure to keep that in check.

Herbs and Spices

What to eat

- Thyme

- Rosemary
- Cinnamon
- Basil
- Garlic
- Ginger
- Turmeric
- Chili peppers
- Paprika

What not to eat

- Nothing, in particular, to be aware of.

Animal and Fish Products

What to eat

- Oily fish, such as herring
- Salmon
- Tuna
- Mackerel
- Sardines
- Lean meats, such as chicken breast/fat-free lean beef

What not to eat

- Make sure to avoid processed meats, such as sausages, since they contain a good amount of nitrates.

Fats

What to eat

- Coconut oil
- Avocado oil
- Olive oil
- Almond butter/oil
- Pine nuts
- Pistachios
- Walnuts
- Cocoa
- Chocolates

What not to eat

- Fried foods
- Vegetable oil

- Soybean oil
- Margarine
- Shortening
- Lard
- Whole milk
- Dairy butter
- Low fat butter

Drinks

What to eat

- Green tea
- Healthy Smoothies
- Red wine is a very moderate amount

What not to eat

- Sugary beverages
- Excessive alcohol

Carbohydrates

What to eat

- Unrefined whole grains
- Whole wheat bread
- Brown rice
- Oatmeal

What not to eat

- Refined carbs
- Pastries
- White bread
- French fries
- Artificial sugar

Can a Vegetarian Diet Reduce Inflammation?

As of recent years, both the Vegan and Vegetarian diets have gained a significant amount of popularity. More and more people are jumping on the bandwagon with each passing day.

A balanced and well-prepared vegan/vegetarian diet does not only help reduce various cardiovascular diseases, but it has also been seen to reduce chronic inflammation.

Various symptoms, such as asthma, inflammatory bowel disease and arthritis, caused by chronic inflammation, are helped with a vegan/vegetarian diet.

The diet's effectiveness can be enhanced even further if you combine a vegan/vegetarian food list. The anti-inflammatory food list is provided in this book. That way, you will be able to bring the best of both worlds.

Anti-Inflammatory Diet Tips

Even if you follow a complete Anti-Inflammatory diet, the following steps will help you up-the-ante and improve your condition.

- Make sure to eat a wide variety of different fruits and vegetables of different colors.
- Make sure to reduce the junk foods that you eat.
- Make sure to eliminate any kind of sugary beverages and sodas from your diet.
- Try to make shopping lists that are packed with healthy meals and snacks that you can munch on for convenience.
- Make sure to always carry a small portion of anti-inflammatory snack while you are on the go.
- Make sure to keep drinking more water.
- Make sure to keep your food intake under your daily calorie intake.
- Try to add Omega-3 supplements and turmeric to your diet.
- Make sure to avoid inactivity and exercise regularly.
- And finally, always make sure to get proper sleep!

These will help you to significantly accelerate your progress.

That being said, I do believe that before moving forward, you should have a good idea of what inflammation actually is. Therefore, the next chapter will focus on giving you a basic insight into the concept of inflammation.

Chapter 2: Looking a Little Bit Into Inflammation

Now that you have a good idea about the Inflammatory Diet, I strongly believe that you should have a good idea of inflammation basics. It will better help you understand what's causing your ailments.

What is Inflammation?

In the simplest terms, inflammation is the process of how the body's immune system reacts whenever it detects the presence of a foreign entity inside the body or any form of injury. During an inflammatory response, white blood cells, alongside several different substances, try to protect the body from further damage that might result from the contamination.

However, things change when this very action takes a turn for the worst.

Whenever you are dealing with arthritis, which is also related to chronic inflammation, the defense mechanism of the body seems to malfunction and trigger an inflammatory response, even though there is no contamination.

Diseases that tend to do these are largely known as "Auto-Immune" diseases, and instead of protecting the body, the body's own auto-immune system starts to harm itself and damage the tissues.

That being said, let's have a look at some of the main reasons for inflammation.

How Inflammation Begins and Proceeds

Before going into details, let me start the book by sharing how "Inflammation" actually works and why you should be concerned.

So, to fully appreciate the situation and severity of the concept, you must understand how inflammation acts.

Whenever your body gets hurt, it automatically creates a response to the injury by sending out specialized agents or "Cells" designated to fend off the invading toxins and other organisms that may have entered.

These cells prepare pathways for fighter cells to attack and completely engulf the attackers.

Once that has happened, another group of cells signals the body and let it know that the fighter cells have accomplished their task. The body is allowed to stop the production of preparatory and fighter cells.

These outcomes are generally responsible for cleaning up any leftover fighter cells and repair the damage dealt.

To keep things simple, there are two responses to such an event:

- Anti-Inflammatory
- Pro-Inflammatory

Each cell involved in the pro stage builds upon the previous cells' work and helps make the immune reaction stronger for any upcoming attack.

During the pro period, symptoms such as redness, swelling itching are common.

Anti-inflammatory is the reverse of pro-inflammatory, and it works to reduce the effects of inflammation.

Several different substances used to block inflammation are made from various essential fatty acids, which the body cannot create independently.

Such acids are required to be acquired through supplements or food.

Just to give you an example, Omega 6 tends to contribute to the increase in inflammation. At the same time, Omega 3 reduces it.

You should keep in mind that the process that I shared above is a very simple and over-simplified version of the whole mechanism. There's a lot more than this, but it should give you a general idea.

There are various substances that play a deeper role in the whole infrastructure that allows the body to control its inflammatory mechanism.

Some of the crucial ones are:

- **Histamine:** White blood cells near the injury site tend to release a substance known as histamine. This helps to increase the permeability of blood vessels around the wound that allows for greater blood flow. This helps to signal the fighter cells and other required substances that regulate the immune response, alerting them to come to the injury site. Histamine also causes redness and swelling around the affected region and results in itchy eyes, rash and runny nose, etc.

- **Cytokines:** These are proteins activated by pro-inflammatory eicosanoids to signal fighter cells to gather at the injury site. They are responsible for diverting energy from the body to catalyst the healing process. The release of this substance tends to cause tiredness and decrease appetite.

- **C-Reactive Protein:** Now, let's talk a bit about Cytokines. Now Cytokines, alongside the other pro-inflammatory eicosanoids, are very closely involved in the activation of a substance known as "C-Reactive Protein." In the simplest terms, the C-Reactive Protein is a specific organic compound produced by the liver in response to messages sent out by the white blood cell near the injury site. These proteins bind themselves to the injury site and act as a watchtower that helps the body identify invading bodies.

- **Leukocytes:** Several types of leukocytes (also known as white blood cells) are critical to the process of neutralizing invading substances. For example, Neutrophils are small and agile and can first arrive at the crime scene to ingest small microbes. However, large substances, such as Macrophages, are required to tackle a large number of microbes.

There are a few more that you should know about, but the core concept remains the same. Whenever your body starts to suffer from an out of control inflammation attack, the action of these and other similar substances tend to go out of control, which ultimately results in very uncomfortable effects.

What Causes Inflammation?

Various factors come into play when considering the reasons as to "What" causes inflammation in a human being. More often than not, the vast majority of reasons are directly linked to poor lifestyle choices. However, it should be noted that aging is a big factor here, as well.

Some of the most crucial causes to know about include:

Aging

The natural process of aging contributes to inflammation, as well. As we age, few of our cells tend to regenerate. Most of them start to die, leaving behind waste materials that tend to trigger inflammation.

Obesity and Inactivity

Excessive inactivity can and will often lead to obesity, which itself is a major cause of inflammation.

Adipose tissue, the layer of fat found right under our skin, is actually responsible for much more than just keeping it warm.

It is a metabolically active layer that causes the body to change the body chemistry and is also affected by the body's other systems.

The fat layer contains many white blood cells and a greater number of fat (obviously).

However, the cell count is actually linked together. Meaning, the more fat there is, the greater number of white cells will be present.

These cells often release pro-inflammatory substances that gradually contribute to the rise of inflammatory effects.

Diet

If we compare, we would soon see that most of the causes of inflammation are related to diet, so we are keeping this on the top of the list.

Harmful substances, such as refined fats, animal products, and refined carbohydrates, tend to do a lot of damage in the long run.

It should be noted, though, that carbohydrates don't directly contribute to inflammation. Refined foods with higher concentration and fats are found to be naturally dense with inflammation, causing substances that affect that gut, increasing inflammation.

The types of fat an individual consumes also play a greater role here. Back in the early days, when everything was simple, people used to stay on a very well-balanced diet on both Omega 3 and Omega 6 fats. However, modern diets tend to have a very high concentration of Omega -6 fat as opposed to Omega 3 fat; this increases the possibility of suffering from inflammation by 10-20%!

The body needs to have a good supply of Omega-3 fatty acids because Omega 6 and Omega 3 compete for the same COX enzymes needed to build large fatty molecules.

COX-2 enzyme, in particular, is essential for making inflammatory prostaglandins.

Too much Omega-6 fatty acids will result in the domination of this enzyme. The body won't be able to utilize these enzymes anymore in conjunction with Omega-3 fats to reduce inflammation.

Nowadays, fats are even chemically modified, and this plays a greater role in inflammation as well. They are made to be more inexpensive, which results in the production of highly inflammatory products.

Stress

Cortisol is a hormone produced by adrenal glands and manages the body's response to stress.

It helps to stimulate a burst of energy and suppresses the action of pro-inflammatory substances.

This also helps to reduce stress by counteracting the effects of pro-inflammatory eicosanoids. However, If you stress too much, the amount of cortisol might increase to a dramatic level, causing your immune cells to lose sensitivity to this hormone and trigger inflammation.

Smoking

Exposure to various toxins, such as cigarette smoke, plays a great role in inflammation. Either secondhand or firsthand, inhaled tobacco tends to extensively cripple the body's capacity to fight diseases by suppressing the production of white blood cells.

So, it's best to avoid smoking as much as possible.

Some Commonly Asked Questions

Should I Detox Before Anti-Inflammation?

When you are detoxing your body, you are essentially flushing out all of the harmful toxins accumulated in your body.

Doing subtle detox before embarking on your Anti-Inflammation diet is an excellent way of ensuring that your diet's effectiveness is accelerated by a lot.

Should I See a Doctor for My Inflammation?

An Anti-Inflammation diet is a diet that is largely based on vegetables and requires an individual to omit certain products like dairy products, such as milk, cheese, and even red meats! Suppose you are already following a similar kind of diet (such as a Vegan Diet). In that case, you should not worry about it that much since your body is already familiar with the change.

However, suppose you are taking such a step for the first time and are trying to completely shift your lifestyle. In that case, it is highly recommended that you consult your physician to ensure that everything is fine.

Alternatively, suppose you are already suffering from an auto-immune disease. In that case, it is even more advisable to consult with your doctor to create a meal plan according to your requirements.

Should I Take More Exercise?

Having a fit and healthy body definitely helps to trim down the possibility of suffering from auto-immune diseases. If you are obese, you might face some serious inflammatory reactions, so it is better to include a minimum exercise regime level in your day-to-day routine.

Chapter 3: One Day Sample Menu

Meal	Meal Name	Ingredients	Nutritional Values
Breakfast	Morning Scrambled Turkey Eggs	• 1 tablespoon coconut oil • 1 medium red bell pepper, diced • ½ medium yellow onion, diced • ¼ teaspoon hot pepper sauce • 3 large free-range eggs • ¼ teaspoon black pepper, freshly ground • ¼ teaspoon salt	• Calories: 435 • Fat: 30g • Carbohydrates: 34g • Protein: 16g
Lunch	Mushroom Pizza	• ¾ pound Portobello mushrooms, stems removed • ½ cup tomato puree • 2 tablespoons olive oil • 2 cloves garlic, minced • ½ cup cashew cheese • Salt and pepper, to taste	• Calories: 112 • Fat: 7g • Carbohydrates: 7g • Protein: 7g
Dinner			
Snack	Coconut Cookies	• ¾ cup of coconut flour • 2 cups of smooth cashew butter • ½ cup of pure maple syrup • 1-2 tablespoon of sprinkles	• Calories: 110 • Fat: 2g • Carbohydrates: 4g • Protein: 18g
Smoothie	Apple and Berry Packed Smoothie	• 2 cups frozen blackberries • ½ cup apple cider • 1 apple, cubed • 2/3 cup non-fat lemon yogurt	• Calories: 200 • Fat: 10g • Carbohydrates: 14g • Protein 2g

Chapter 4: Breakfast Recipes

Coconut and Cinnamon Bowl

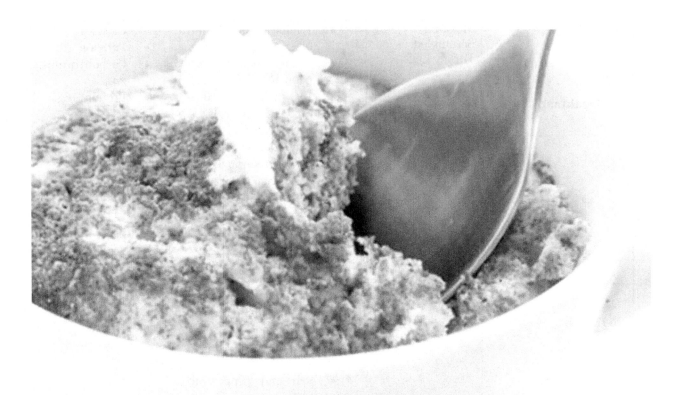

Serving: 4

Prep Time: 5 minutes

Cook Time: 5 minutes

<u>Ingredients</u>

- 1 cup of water
- 1/2 cup cashew cream
- ½ cup of unsweetened dried coconut, shredded
- 1 tablespoon of oat bran
- 1 tablespoon of flaxseed meal

- 1/2 tablespoon of almond butter
- 1 ½ teaspoons of stevia
- ½ teaspoon of cinnamon
- Toppings, such as blueberries or banana slices

How To

1. Add the ingredients mentioned above to a small pot, mix well until fully incorporated.
2. Transfer the pot to your stove over medium-low heat and bring the mix to a slow boil.
3. Stir well and remove the heat.
4. Divide the mixture into equal servings and let them sit for 10 minutes.
5. Top with your desired toppings and enjoy!

Nutrition Values (Per Serving)

- Calories: 171
- Fat: 16g
- Protein: 2g
- Carbohydrates: 8g

Walnut and Banana Bowl

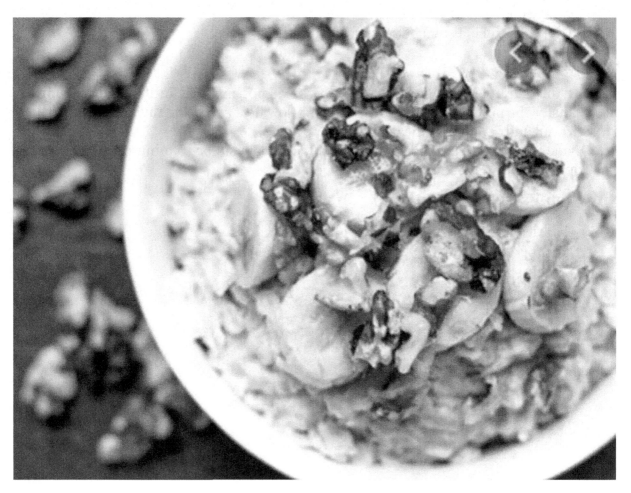

Serving: 4

Prep Time: 10 minutes

Cook Time: 15 minutes

Ingredients

- 2 cups of water
- 1 cup steel-cut oats
- 1 cup almond milk
- ¼ cup walnuts, chopped
- 2 tablespoons chia seeds
- 2 bananas, peeled and mashed
- 1 teaspoon vanilla flavoring

How To

1. Take a pot and add all ingredients, toss well.

2. Bring it to simmer over medium heat.

3. Let it cook for 15 minutes, divide amongst the bowl.

4. Enjoy!

Nutrition Values (Per Serving)

- Calories: 162
- Fat: 4g
- Carbohydrates: 11g
- Protein: 4g

Amazing Pesto Egg

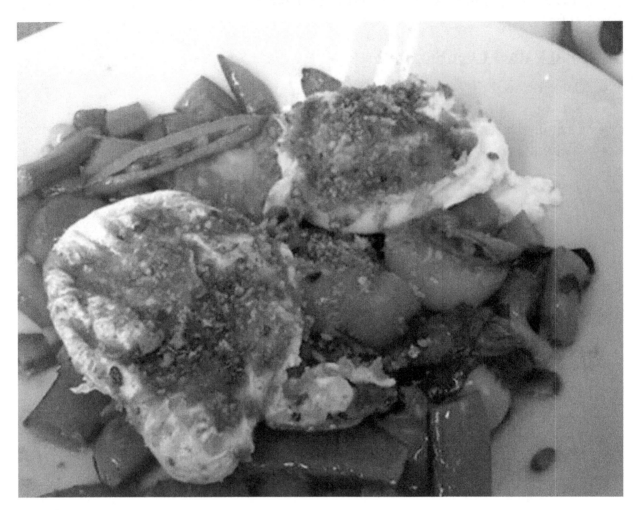

Serving: 2

Prep Time: 5 minutes

Cook Time: 5 minutes

Ingredients

- 2 large whole eggs
- 1/2 tablespoon almond butter
- 1/2 tablespoon pesto
- 1 tablespoon creamed coconut almond milk
- Sunflower seeds and pepper as needed

How To

1. Take a bowl and crack open your egg.

2. Season with a pinch of sunflower seeds and pepper.

3. Pour eggs into a pan.
4. Add almond butter and introduce heat.
5. Cook on low heat and gently add pesto.
6. Once the egg is cooked and scrambled, remove heat.
7. Spoon in coconut cream and mix well.
8. Turn on the heat and cook on LOW for a while until you have a creamy texture.
9. Serve and enjoy!

Nutrition Values (Per Serving)

- Calories: 467
- Fat: 41g
- Carbohydrates: 3g
- Protein: 20g

Perfect Barley Porridge

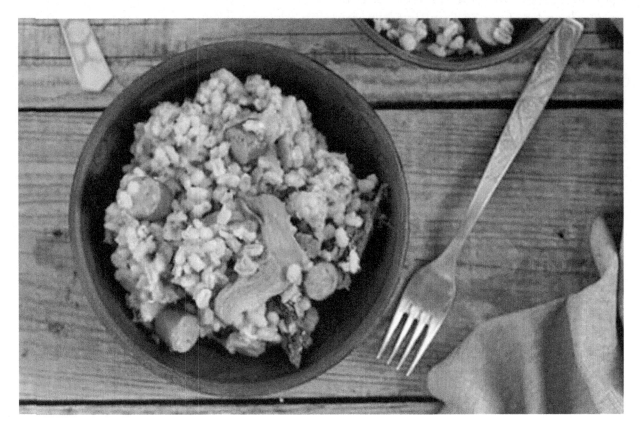

Serving: 4

Prep Time: 5 minutes

Cook Time: 25 minutes

Ingredients

- 1 cup barley
- 1 cup of wheat berries
- 2 cups unsweetened almond milk
- 2 cups of water
- Toppings, such as hazelnuts, honey, berry, etc.

How To

1. Take a medium saucepan and place it over medium-high heat.
2. Place barley, almond milk, wheat berries, water and bring to a boil.
3. Reduce the heat to low and simmer for 25 minutes.
4. Divide amongst serving bowls and top with your desired toppings.
5. Serve and enjoy!

Nutrition Values (Per Serving)

- Calories: 295
- Fat: 8g
- Carbohydrates: 56g
- Protein: 6g

Morning Scrambled Turkey Eggs

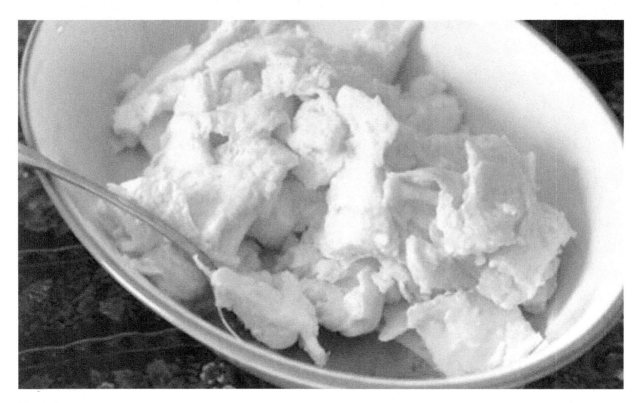

Serving: 2

Prep Time: 15 minutes

Cook Time: 15 minutes

Ingredients

- 1 tablespoon coconut oil
- 1 medium red bell pepper, diced
- ½ medium yellow onion, diced
- ¼ teaspoon hot pepper sauce
- 3 large free-range eggs
- ¼ teaspoon black pepper, freshly ground
- ¼ teaspoon salt

How To

1. Set a pan to medium-high heat and add coconut oil; let it heat up.

2. Add onions and sauté.

3. Add turkey and red pepper.

4. Cook until turkey is cooked.

5. Take a bowl and beat eggs, stir in salt and pepper.

6. Pour eggs in the pan with turkey and gently cook and scramble eggs.

7. Top with hot sauce and enjoy!

Nutrition Values (Per Serving)

- Calories: 435
- Fat: 30g
- Carbohydrates: 34g
- Protein: 16g

Lovely Pumpkin Oats

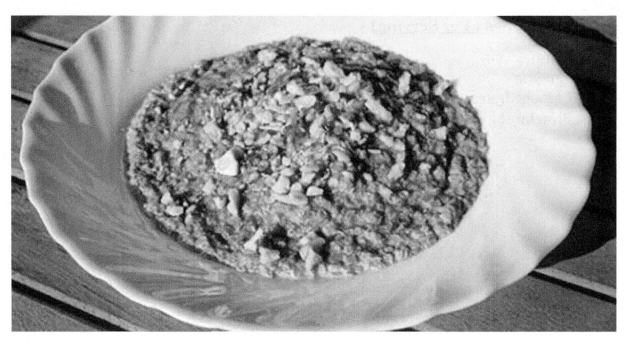

Serving: 3

Prep Time: 5 minutes

Cook Time: 8 minutes

Ingredients

- 1 cup quick-cooking rolled oats
- ¾ cup almond milk
- ½ cup canned pumpkin puree
- ¼ teaspoon pumpkin pie spice
- 1 teaspoon ground cinnamon

How To

1. Take a safe microwave bowl and add oats, almond milk, and microwave on high for 1-2 minutes.
2. Add more almond milk if needed to achieve your desired consistency.
3. Cook for 30 seconds more.
4. Stir in pumpkin puree, pumpkin pie spice, ground cinnamon.
5. Heat gently and enjoy!

Nutrition(Per Serving)

- Calories: 229
- Fat: 4g

- Carbohydrates: 38g
- Protein:10g

Zucchini and Carrot Combo

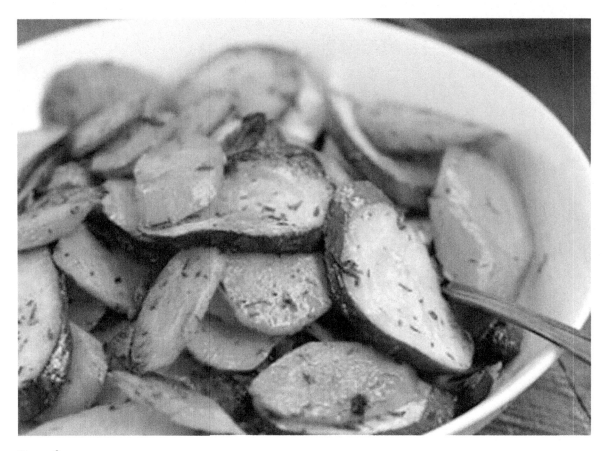

Serving: 3

Prep Time: 10 minutes

Cook Time: 8 hours

Ingredients

- ½ cup steel cut oats
- 1 cup of coconut milk
- 1 carrot, grated
- ¼ zucchini, grated
- Pinch of nutmeg
- ½ teaspoon cinnamon powder
- 2 tablespoons brown sugar
- ¼ cup pecans, chopped

How To

1. Grease the Slow Cooker well.

2. Add oats, zucchini, milk, carrot, nutmeg, cloves, sugar, cinnamon, and stir well.

3. Place lid and cook on LOW for 8 hours.

4. Divide amongst serving bowls and enjoy!

Nutrition Values (Per Serving)

- Calories: 200
- Fat: 4g
- Carbohydrates: 11g
- Protein: 5g

Herb and Avocado Omelet

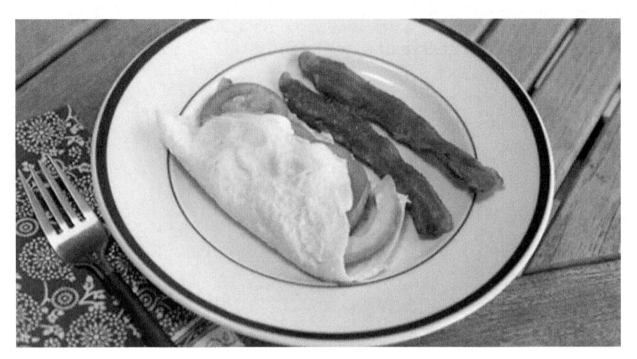

Serving: 2

Prep Time: 2 minutes

Cook Time: 10 minutes

Ingredients

- 3 large free-range eggs
- ½ medium avocado, sliced
- ½ cup almonds, sliced
- Salt and pepper as needed

How To

1. Take a non-stick skillet and place it over medium-high heat.
2. Take a bowl and add eggs, beat the eggs.
3. Pour into the skillet and cook for 1 minute.
4. Lower heat to low and cook for 4 minutes.
5. Top the omelet with almonds and avocado.
6. Sprinkle salt and pepper and serve.
7. Enjoy!

Nutrition Values (Per Serving)

- Calories: 193

- Fat: 15g
- Carbohydrates: 5g
- Protein: 10g

Tomato Egg Scramble

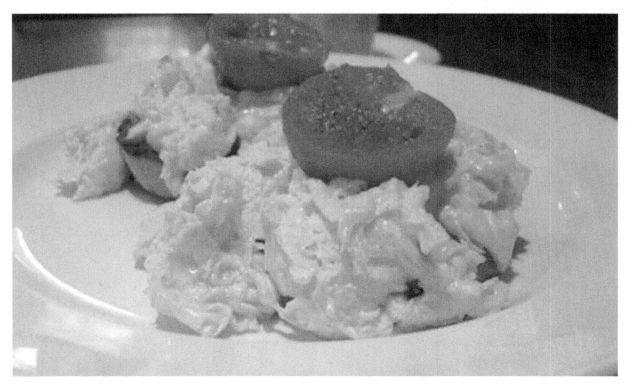

Serving: 2

Prep Time: 10 minutes

Cook Time: 5 minutes

Ingredients

- 2 whole eggs
- ½ cup fresh basil, chopped
- 2 tablespoons olive oil
- ½ teaspoon red pepper flakes, crushed
- 1 cup grape tomatoes, chopped
- Salt and pepper to taste

How To

1. Take a bowl and whisk in eggs, salt, pepper, red pepper flakes and mix well.
2. Add tomatoes, basil, and mix.
3. Take a skillet and place it over medium-high heat.
4. Add egg mixture and cook for 5 minutes and cooked and scrambled.
5. Enjoy!

Nutrition Values (Per Serving)

- Calories: 130
- Fat: 10g
- Carbohydrates: 8g
- Protein: 1.8g

Choco-Nana Pancakes

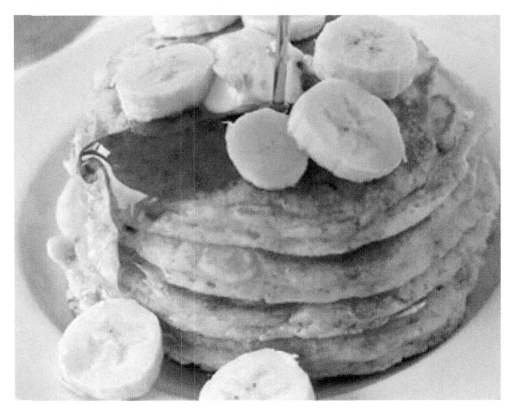

Serving: 2

Prep Time: 5 minutes

Cook Time: 6 minutes

Ingredients

- 2 large eggs, pasture-raised
- 2 large bananas, peeled and mashed
- 1 teaspoon pure vanilla extract
- 2 tablespoons almond butter
- 3 tablespoons cacao powder
- 1/8 teaspoon salt
- Coconut oil, for greasing

How To

1. Take a skillet and preheat on medium-low heat.
2. Grease the pan with coconut oil.
3. Add all ingredients to a food processor and blend until smooth.
4. Pour the batter into a skillet and make the pancake.
5. Cook for 3 minutes on each side.

6. Serve and enjoy!

Nutrition Values (Per Serving)

- Calories: 303
- Fat: 17g
- Carbohydrates: 36g
- Protein: 5g

Awesome Breakfast Parfait

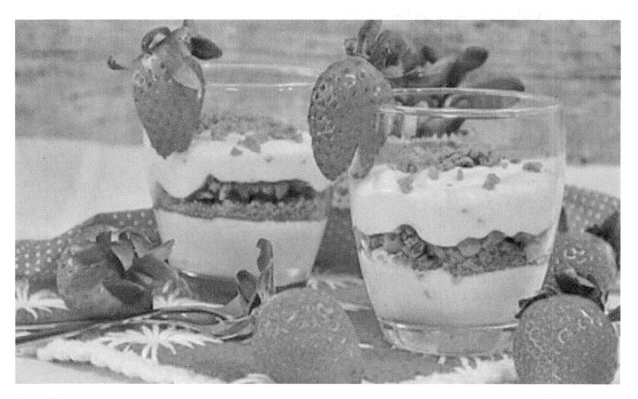

Serving: 2

Prep Time: 5 minutes

Cook Time: Nil

Ingredients

- 1 teaspoon sunflower seeds
- ½ cup low-fat milk
- 1 cup all-purpose flour
- 1 teaspoon vanilla
- 3 eggs, beaten
- 1 teaspoon baking soda
- 2 cups non-fat Greek yogurt

How To

1. Break up pretzels into small-sized portions and slice up the strawberries.

2. Add yogurt to the bottom of the glass and top with pretzels pieces and strawberries.

3. Add more yogurt and keep repeating until you have used up all ingredients.

4. Enjoy!

Nutrition Values (Per Serving)

- Calorie: 304
- Fat: 1g
- Carbohydrates: 58g
- Protein: 15g

Healthy Zucchini Stir Fry

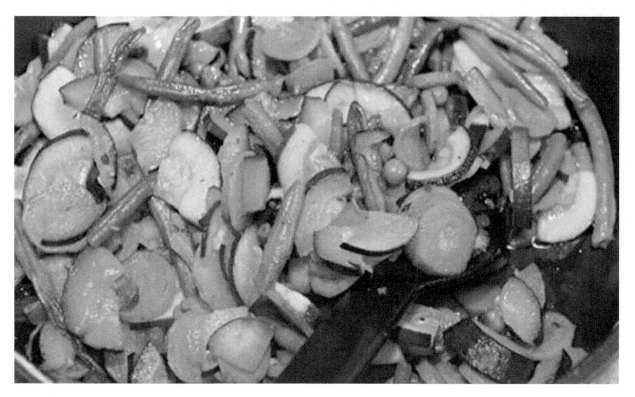

Serving: 4

Prep Time: 10 minutes

Cook Time: 10 minutes

Ingredients

- 2 tablespoons of heaping olive oil
- 1 whole medium-sized onion, sliced thinly
- 2 whole medium-sized zucchini, cut up into thin sized strips
- 2 heaping tablespoons of flavored teriyaki sauce, low sodium
- 1 whole tablespoon of coconut aminos
- 1 whole tablespoon of a sesame seed, toasted
- Ground pepper (black) as much as needed

How To

1. Take a skillet and place it over medium level heat.
2. Add onions and stir cook for 5 minutes.
3. Add your zucchini and stir cook for 1 minute more.
4. Gently add the sauces alongside the sesame seeds.
5. Cook for 5 minutes more until the zucchini are soft.

6. Finally, add in pepper and enjoy!

<u>Nutrition Values (Per Serving)</u>

- Calories: 110
- Fat: 9g
- Carbohydrates: 8g
- Protein: 3g

Turmeric Protein Donuts

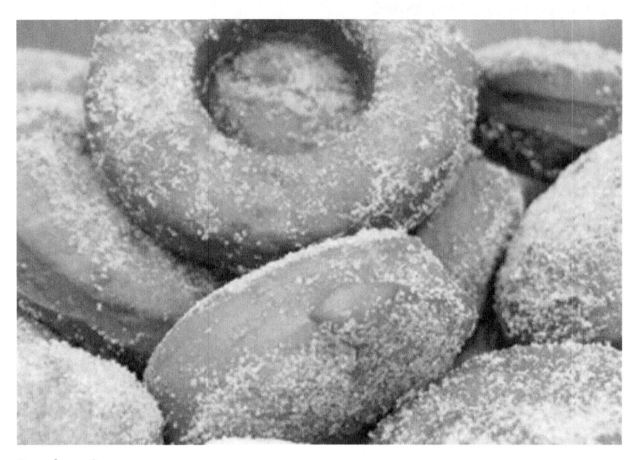

Serving: 8

Prep Time: 50 minutes

Cook Time: 0 minutes

Ingredients

- 1 ½ cups cashews, raw
- 2 tablespoons maple syrup
- ¼ teaspoon vanilla extract
- 1 tablespoon vanilla protein powder
- ½ cup Medjool dates pitted
- ¼ cup dark chocolate
- ½ cup coconut, shredded
- 1 teaspoon turmeric powder

How To

1. Add all ingredients except chocolate to a food processor.
2. Pulse until smooth.

3. Roll batter 8 balls and press into silicone mold.
4. Place into the refrigerator for 30 minutes.
5. Make the chocolate topping.
6. Once done, remove the donuts from the mold.
7. Then drizzle with chocolate.
8. Serve and enjoy!

Nutrition Values (Per Serving)

- Calories: 320
- Fat: 26g
- Carbohydrates: 20g
- Protein: 11g

Savory Pancake Blast

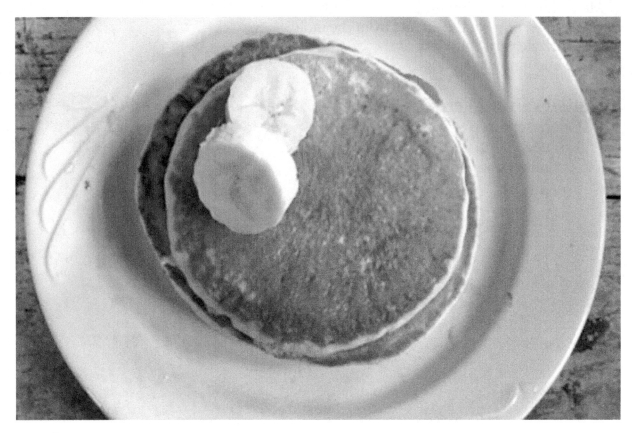

Serving: 4

Prep Time: 5 minutes

Cook Time: 6 minutes

Ingredients

- ¼ teaspoon turmeric powder
- 1 cup of coconut milk
- ½ cup tapioca flour
- ½ cup almond flour
- 1 red onion, chopped
- 1 cilantro leaves, chopped
- ½ inch ginger, chopped
- 1 teaspoon salt
- ¼ teaspoon black pepper, ground

How To

1. Take a bowl and mix all ingredients until well-combined.
2. Heat a pan on low, medium heat and grease with oil.
3. Pour ¼ cup batter onto the pan and spread the mixture to create a pancake.

4. Fry 3 minutes for each side.
5. Repeat the process.
6. Serve and enjoy!

<u>Nutrition Values (Per Serving)</u>

- Calories: 340
- Fat: 30g
- Carbohydrates: 40g
- Protein: 17g

Banana Steel Oats

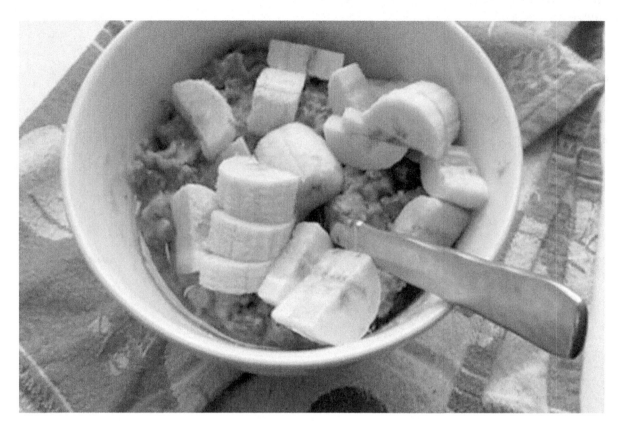

Serving: 3

Prep Time: 10 minutes

Cook Time: 15 minutes

Ingredients

- 1 small banana
- 1 cup almond milk
- ¼ teaspoon cinnamon, ground
- ½ cup rolled oats
- 1 tablespoon honey

How To

1. Take a saucepan and add half the banana, whisk in almond milk, ground cinnamon.
2. Season with sunflower seeds.
3. Stir until the banana is mashed well, bring the mixture to a boil and stir in oats.
4. Lower heat to medium-low and simmer for 5-7 minutes until the oats are tender.
5. Dice the remaining half of banana and top oatmeal.
6. Enjoy!

Nutrition(Per Serving)

- Calories: 358
- Fat: 6g
- Carbohydrates: 76g
- Protein: 7g

Blue Cheese, Fig and Arugula Salad

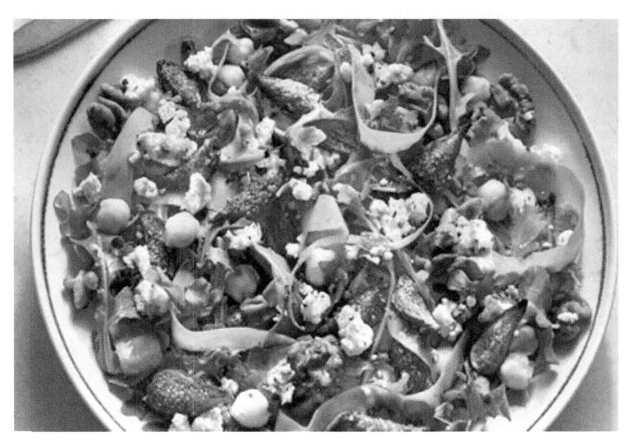

Serving: 4

Prep Time: 10 minutes

Cook Time: 0 minutes

Ingredients

- ¼ cup cashew cheese
- 2 bags arugula
- 1-pint figs, quartered
- 3 tablespoons balsamic vinegar
- 3 tablespoons olive oil
- 1 teaspoon Dijon mustard
- Salt and pepper, to taste

How To

1. Take a bowl and add Dijon mustard, balsamic, vinegar, olive oil, salt, and pepper.
2. Whisk them thoroughly, then set aside for 30 minutes to marinate.
3. Take 4 serving plates and add cheese and figs on top.
4. Drizzle with 1 ½ tablespoons for each.

5. Serve and enjoy!

Nutrition Values (Per Serving)

- Calories: 143
- Fat: 13g
- Carbohydrates: 5g
- Protein: 3g

Quinoa and Cinnamon Bowl

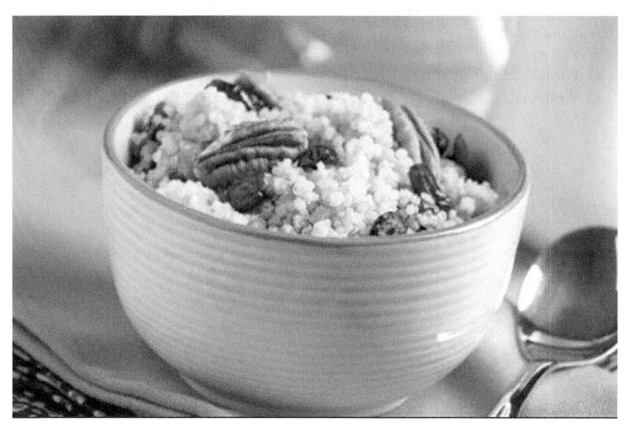

Serving: 2

Prep Time: 10 minutes

Cook Time: 15 minutes

Ingredients

- 1 cup uncooked quinoa
- 1 ½ cups of water
- ½ teaspoon ground cinnamon
- ½ teaspoon sunflower seeds
- A drizzle of almond/coconut milk for serving

How To

1. Rinse quinoa thoroughly underwater.
2. Take a medium-sized saucepan and add quinoa, water, cinnamon, and seeds.
3. Stir and place it over medium-high heat.
4. Bring the mix to a boil.
5. Reduce heat to low and simmer for 10 minutes.
6. Once cooked, remove from the heat and let it cool.

7. Serve with a drizzle of almond or coconut milk.
8. Enjoy!

Nutrition Values (Per Serving)

- Calories: 255
- Fat: 13g
- Carbohydrates: 33g
- Protein: 5g

Hearty Pineapple Oatmeal

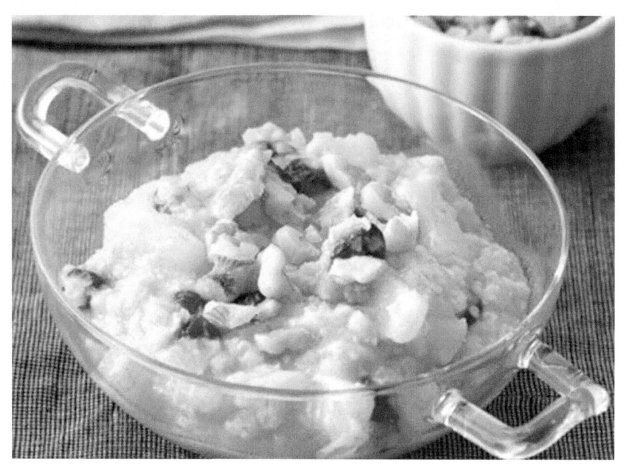

Serving: 5

Prep Time: 10 minutes

Cook Time: 4-8 hours

Ingredients

- 1 cup steel-cut oats
- 4 cups unsweetened almond milk
- 2 medium apples, slashed
- 1 teaspoon coconut oil
- 1 teaspoon cinnamon
- ¼ teaspoon nutmeg
- 2 tablespoons maple syrup, unsweetened
- A drizzle of lemon juice

How To

1. Add listed ingredients to a cooking pan and mix well.

2. Cook on very low flame for 8 hours or on high flame for 4 hours.

3. Gently stir.

4. Add toppings your desired toppings.

5. Serve and enjoy!

6. Store in the fridge for later use; make sure to add a splash of almond milk after re-heating for added flavor.

Nutrition Values (Per Serving)

- Calories: 180
- Fat: 5g
- Carbohydrates: 31g
- Protein: 5g

Avocado Egg

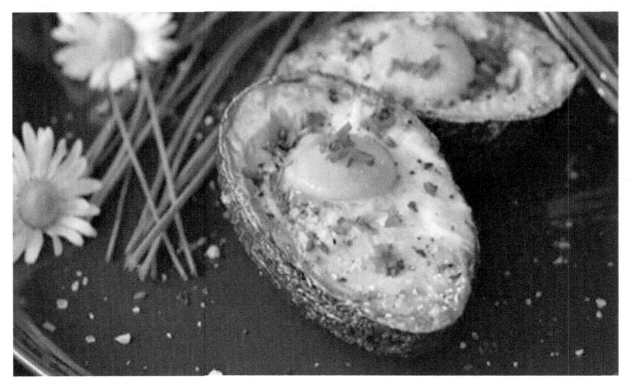

Serving: 1

Prep Time: 5 minutes

Cook Time: 20 minutes

Ingredients

- 2 ripe avocados
- 4 eggs
- Salt
- Pepper, to taste

How To

1. Preheat the oven to 350 degrees F.
2. Slice the avocado and remove the seed.
3. Crack one egg into the hollow depression of the avocado where the seed has been.
4. Season with salt and pepper to taste.
5. Bake in the oven for 20 minutes.
6. Serve and enjoy!

Nutrition Values (Per Serving)

- Calories: 290

- Fat: 24g
- Carbohydrates: 10g
- Protein: 11g

Swiss Chard Omelet

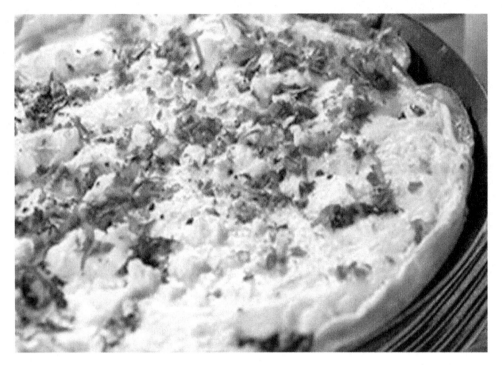

Serving: 2

Prep Time: 5 minutes

Cook Time: 5 minutes

Ingredients

- 2 eggs, lightly beaten
- 2 cups Swiss chard, sliced
- 1 tablespoon almond butter
- ½ teaspoon sunflower seeds
- Fresh pepper

How To

1. Take a non-stick frying pan and place it over medium-low heat.
2. Once the almond butter melts, add Swiss chard and stir cook for 2 minutes.
3. Pour egg into the pan and gently stir them into the Swiss chard.
4. Season with garlic, sunflower seeds, and pepper.
5. Cook for 2 minutes.
6. Serve and enjoy!

Nutrition Values (Per Serving)

- Calories: 260

- Fat: 21g
- Carbohydrates: 4g
- Protein: 14g

Chapter 5: Lunch Recipes
Mango Chicken Meal

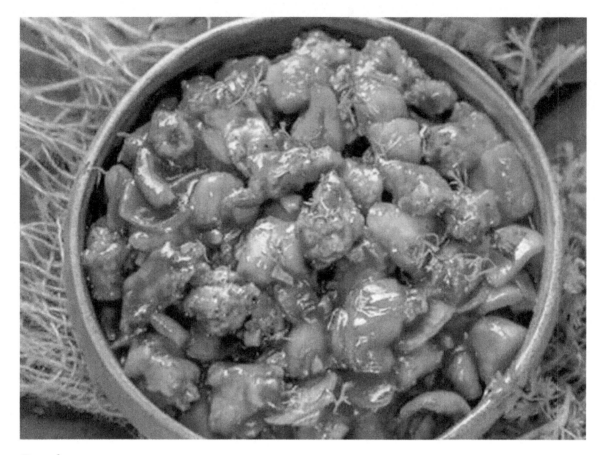

Serving: 4

Prep Time: 25 minutes

Cook Time: 10 minutes

Ingredients

- 2 medium mangoes, peeled and sliced
- 10-ounce coconut almond milk
- 4 teaspoons of vegetable oil
- 4 teaspoons of spicy curry paste
- 14-ounce chicken breast halves, skinless and boneless, cut into cubes
- 4 medium shallots
- 1 large English cucumber, sliced and seeded

How To

1. Slice half of the mangoes and add the halves to a bowl.

2. Add mangoes and coconut almond milk to a blender and blend until you have a smooth puree.

3. Keep the mixture on the side.

4. Take a large-sized pot and place it over medium heat, add oil and allow the oil to heat up.

5. Add curry paste and cook for 1 minute until you have a nice fragrance; add shallots and chicken to the pot and cook for 5 minutes.

6. Pour mango puree into the mix and allow it to heat up.

7. Serve the cooked chicken with mango puree and cucumbers.

8. Enjoy!

Nutrition Values (Per Serving)

- Calories: 398
- Fat: 20g
- Carbohydrates: 32g
- Protein: 26g

Roasted Cauliflower

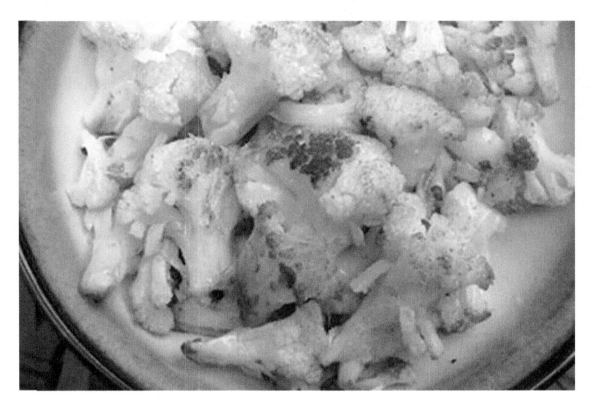

Serving: 8

Prep Time: 5 minutes

Cook Time: 30 minutes

Ingredients

- 1 large cauliflower head
- 2 tablespoons melted coconut oil
- 2 tablespoons fresh thyme
- 1 teaspoon Celtic sea sunflower seeds
- 1 teaspoon fresh ground pepper
- 1 head roasted garlic
- 2 tablespoons fresh thyme for garnish

How To

1. Preheat your oven to 425-degree F.

2. Rinse cauliflower and trim, core and sliced.

3. Lay cauliflower evenly on a rimmed baking tray.

4. Drizzle coconut oil evenly over cauliflower, sprinkle thyme leaves.

5. Season with a pinch of sunflower seeds and pepper.

6. Squeeze roasted garlic.

7. Roast cauliflower until slightly caramelized for about 30 minutes, making sure to turn once.

8. Garnish with fresh thyme leaves.

9. Enjoy!

Nutrition Values (Per Serving)

- Calories: 129
- Fat: 11g
- Carbohydrates: 6g
- Protein: 7g

Asparagus and Walnut Deal

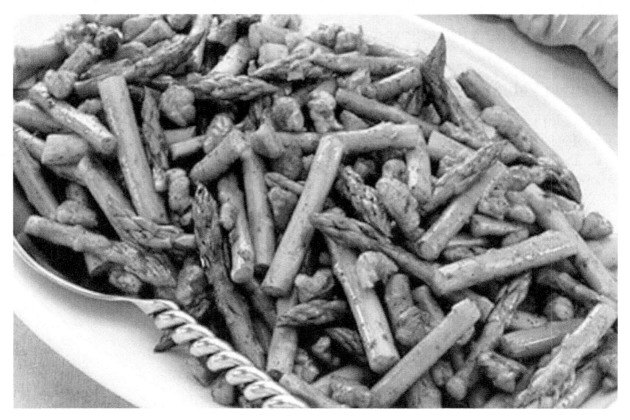

Serving: 4

Prep Time: 5 minutes

Cook Time: 5 minutes

Ingredients

- 1 ½ tablespoons olive oil
- ¾ pound asparagus, trimmed
- ¼ cup walnuts, chopped
- Sunflower seeds and pepper to taste

How To

1. Place a skillet over medium heat, add olive oil and let it heat up.
2. Add asparagus, sauté for 5 minutes until browned.
3. Season with sunflower seeds and pepper.
4. Remove heat.
5. Add walnuts and toss.
6. Serve warm!

Nutrition Values (Per Serving)

- Calories: 124
- Fat: 12g
- Carbohydrates: 2g
- Protein: 3g

Chicken and Carrot Stew

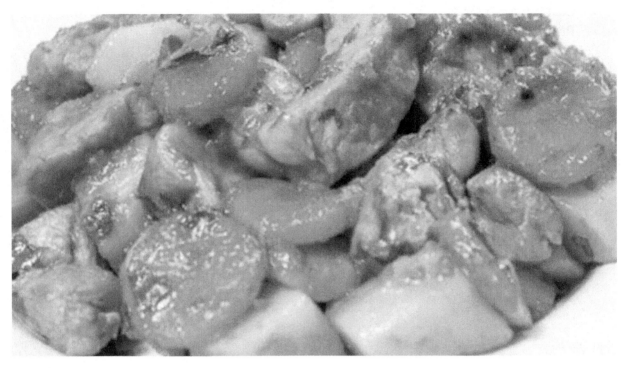

Serving: 4

Prep Time: 15 minutes

Cook Time: 6 hours

Ingredients

- 4 boneless chicken breasts, cubed
- 3 cups of carrots, peeled and cubed
- 1 cup onion, chopped
- 1 cup tomatoes, chopped
- 1 teaspoon of dried thyme
- 2 cups of chicken broth
- 2 garlic cloves, minced
- Sunflower seeds and pepper as needed

How To

1. Add all of the listed Ingredients to a Slow Cooker.

2. Stir and close the lid.

3. Cook for 6 hours.

4. Serve hot and enjoy!

Nutrition Values (Per Serving)

- Calories: 182
- Fat: 3g
- Carbohydrates: 10g
- Protein: 39g

Grilled Chicken and Blueberry Medley

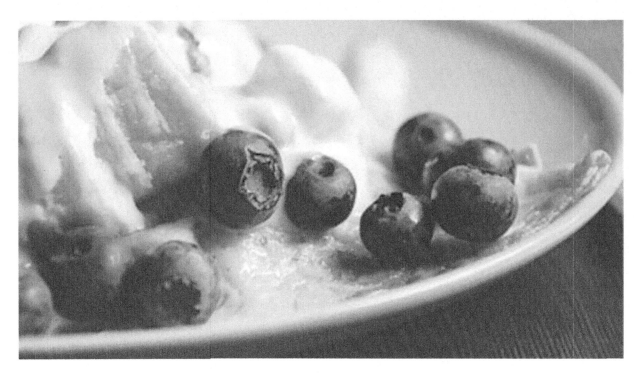

Serving: 5

Prep Time: 10 minutes

Cook Time: 25 minutes

Ingredients

- 5 cups mixed greens
- 1 cup blueberries
- ¼ cup slivered almonds
- 2 cups chicken breasts, cooked and cubed

For dressing

- ¼ cup olive oil
- ¼ cup apple cider vinegar
- ¼ cup blueberries
- 2 tablespoons honey
- Sunflower seeds and pepper to taste

How To

1. Take a bowl and add greens, berries, almonds, chicken cubes and mix well.
2. Take a bowl and mix the dressing ingredients, pour the mix into a blender and blitz until smooth.

3. Add dressing on top of the chicken cubes and toss well.

4. Season more and enjoy it!

Nutrition Values (Per Serving)

- Calories: 266
- Fat: 17g
- Carbohydrates: 18g
- Protein: 10g

Slow-Cooker Cauliflower Mis-Mash

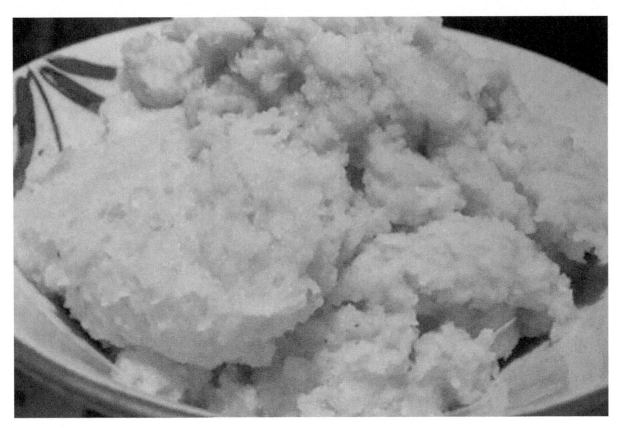

Serving: 6

Prep Time: 10 minutes

Cooking Time: 6 hours

Ingredients:

- 1 cauliflower head, florets separated
- 1/3 cup dill, chopped
- 6 garlic cloves
- 2 tablespoons olive oil
- Pinch of black pepper

How To:

1. Add cauliflower to Slow Cooker.
2. Add dill, garlic, and water to cover them.
3. Place lid and cook on HIGH for 5 hours.
4. Drain the flowers.
5. Season with pepper and add oil, mash using a potato masher.
6. Whisk and serve.

7. Enjoy!

Nutritional Contents:

- Calories: 207
- Fat: 4g
- Carbohydrates: 14g
- Protein: 3g

Sweet Potato Platter

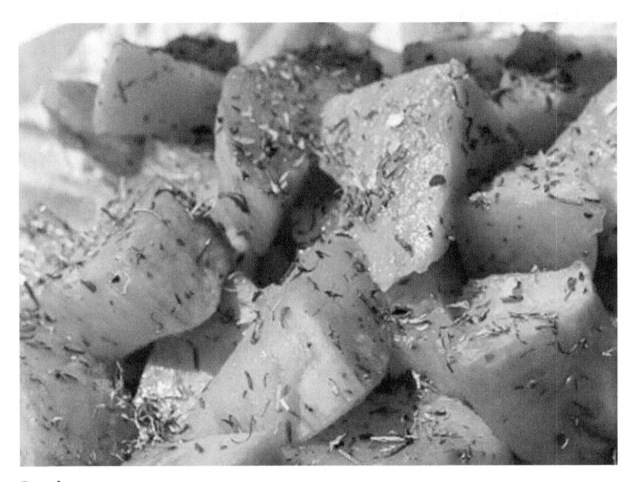

Serving: 4

Prep Time: 5 minutes

Cook Time: 7-8 hours

Ingredients

- 6 sweet potatoes, washed and dried

How To

1. Loosely ball up 7-8 pieces of aluminum foil in the bottom of your Slow Cooker, covering about half of the surface area.
2. Prick each potato 6-8 times using a fork.
3. Wrap each potato with foil and seal them.
4. Place wrapped potatoes in the cooker on top of the foil bed.
5. Place lid and cook on LOW for 7-8 hours.
6. Use tongs to remove the potatoes and unwrap them.
7. Serve and enjoy!

Nutrition Values (Per Serving)

- Calories: 129
- Fat: 0g
- Carbohydrates: 30g
- Protein: 2g

Italian Garlic Scallops

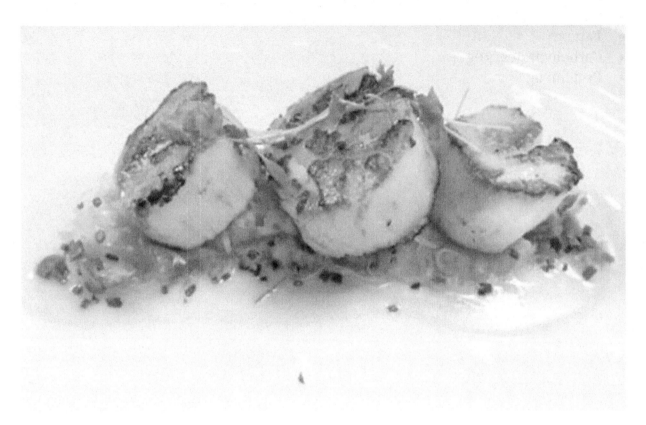

Serving: 4

Prep Time: 5 minutes

Cook Time: 25 minutes

Ingredients

- 8 tablespoons almond butter
- 2 garlic cloves, minced
- 16 large sea scallops
- Salt and pepper to taste
- 1 ½ tablespoons olive oil

How To

1. Season scallops with salt and pepper.
2. Take a skillet and place it over medium heat, add oil and let it heat up.
3. Sauté scallops for 2 minutes per side, repeat until all scallops are cooked.
4. Add butter to the skillet and let it melt.
5. Stir in garlic and cook for 15 minutes.
6. Return scallops to skillet and stir to coat.
7. Serve and enjoy!

Nutrition (Per Serving)

- Calories: 417
- Fat: 31g
- Net Carbohydrates: 5g
- Protein: 29g

Spiced Up Tuna Rolls

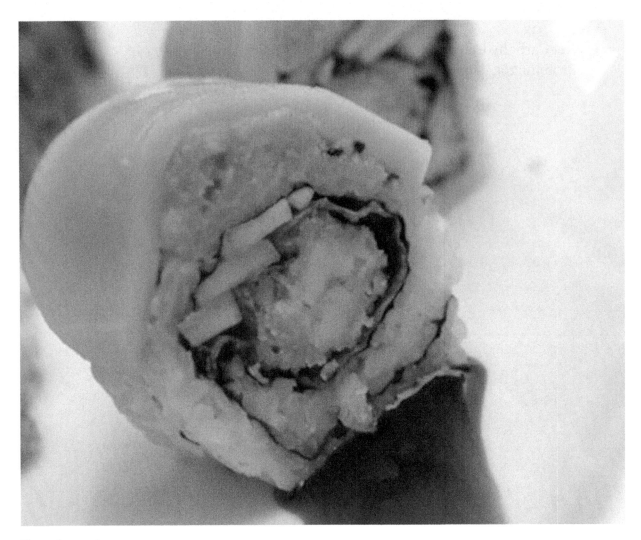

Serving: 6

Prep Time: 10 minutes

Cook Time: 0 minute

Ingredients

- 1 can yellowfin tuna, wild-caught
- 1 medium cucumber
- 2 slices avocado, diced
- 1/8 teaspoon salt
- 1/8 teaspoon pepper

How To

1. Take a cucumber and use a mandolin to thinly slice it lengthwise.

2. Take a mixing bowl and add avocado and tuna.
3. Season with salt and pepper to taste.
4. Spoon the tuna and avocado mixture.
5. Spread it consistently on cucumber slices.
6. Roll the cucumber slices.
7. Use a toothpick to secure the ends.
8. Serve chilled and enjoy!

Nutrition Values (Per Serving)

- Calories: 135
- Fat: 10g
- Carbohydrates: 6g
- Protein: 7g

Spicy Kale Chips

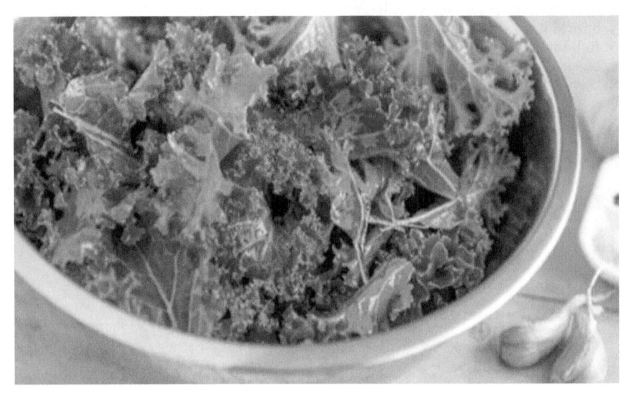

Serving: 4

Prep Time: 10 minutes

Cook Time: 20 minutes

Ingredients

- 1 bunch curly kale, rinsed
- 1/8 teaspoon garlic powder
- ¼ teaspoon salt
- Spray oil for greasing
- ¼ teaspoon cayenne pepper, ground
- 1/8 teaspoon black pepper

How To

1. Preheat your oven to 300 degrees F.
2. Pat dry kale to remove water.
3. Take a baking sheet lined with foil and place torn kale leaves.
4. Spray with cooking oil.
5. Season with garlic powder and black pepper.
6. Bake in your oven for 20 minutes.
7. Serve and enjoy!

Nutrition Values (Per Serving)

- Calories: 5
- Fat: 0.08g
- Carbohydrates: 1g
- Protein: 0.4g

Mushroom Pizza

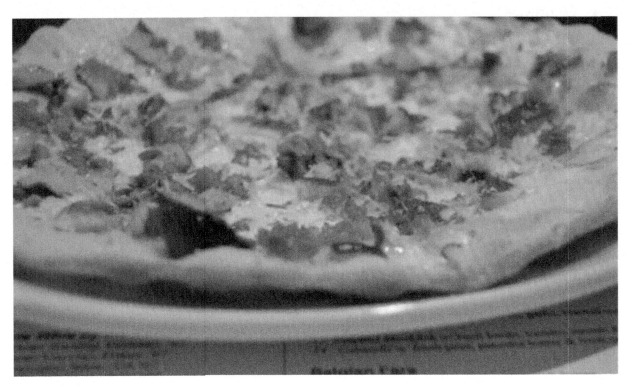

Serving: 4

Prep Time: 10 minutes

Cook Time: 15 minutes

Ingredients

- ¾ pound Portobello mushrooms, stems removed
- ½ cup tomato puree
- 2 tablespoons olive oil
- 2 cloves garlic, minced
- ½ cup cashew cheese
- Salt and pepper, to taste

How To

1. Preheat your oven to 350 degrees F.
2. Brush oil on the inverted side of the mushrooms.
3. Brush with sprinkle garlic and tomato puree, then add cashew cheese on top.
4. Place it on a baking pan.
5. Bake for 15 minutes.
6. Serve and enjoy!

Nutrition Values (Per Serving)

- Calories: 112
- Fat: 7g
- Carbohydrates: 7g
- Protein: 7g

Salty Caramel Dip

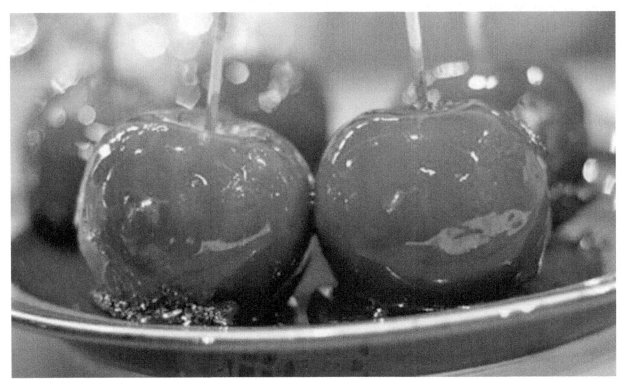

Serving: 2

Prep Time: 5 minutes

Cook Time: 0 minute

Ingredients

- 1 cup soft Medjool dates, pitted
- 1 teaspoon vanilla extract
- ¼ cup almond milk
- 1 teaspoon fresh lemon juice
- 1 tablespoon coconut oil
- ¼ teaspoon salt

How To

1. Add all ingredients to your blender.
2. Pulse until you get a smooth mixture.
3. Serve chilled and enjoy!

Nutrition Values (Per Serving)

- Calories: 113
- Fat: 7.2g

- Carbohydrates: 11.2g
- Protein: 0.4g

Thai Pumpkin Seafood Stew

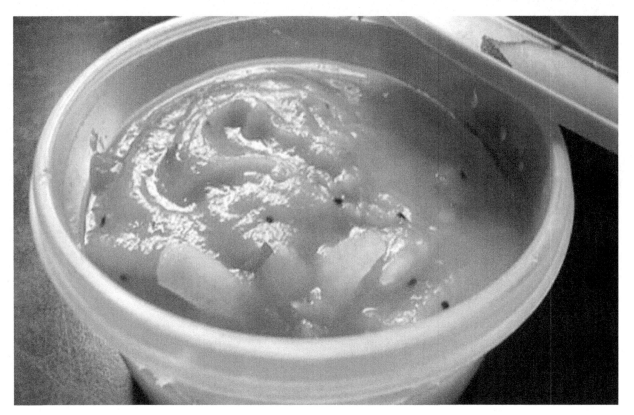

Serving: 4

Prep Time: 5 minutes

Cook Time: 35 minutes

Ingredients

- 1 ½ tablespoons fresh galangal, chopped
- 1 teaspoon lime zest
- 1 small kabocha squash
- 32 medium-sized mussels, fresh
- 1 pound shrimp
- 16 thai leaves
- 1 can coconut milk
- 1 tablespoon lemongrass, minced
- 4 garlic cloves, roughly chopped
- 32 medium clams, fresh
- 1 ½ pounds fresh salmon
- 2 tablespoons coconut oil
- Pepper to taste

How To

1. Add coconut milk, lemongrass, galangal, garlic, lime leaves in a small-sized saucepan, bring to a boil.

2. Let it simmer for 25 minutes.

3. Strain mixture through a fine sieve into the large soup pot and bring to a simmer.

4. Add oil to a pan and heat up; add Kabocha squash.

5. Season with salt and pepper, sauté for 5 minutes.

6. Add mix to coconut mix.

7. Heat oil in a pan and add fish shrimp, season with salt and pepper, cook for 4 minutes.

8. Add mixture to coconut milk mix alongside clams and mussels.

9. Simmer for 8 minutes, garnish with basil and enjoy!

Nutrition Values (Per Serving)

- Calories: 370
- Fat: 16g
- Net Carbohydrates: 10g
- Protein: 16g

Pistachio Sole Fish

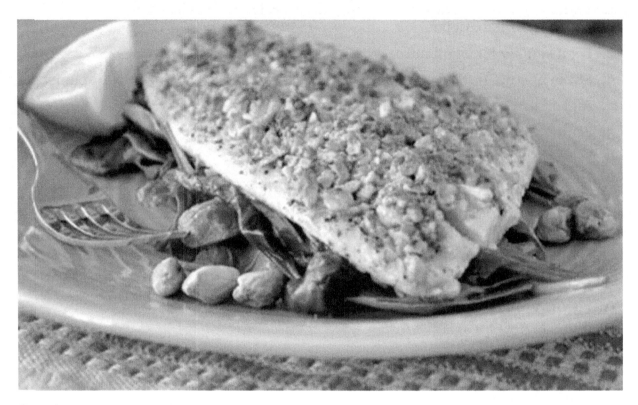

Serving: 4

Prep Time: 5 minutes

Cook Time: 10 minutes

Ingredients

- 4 (5 ounces) boneless sole fillets
- Sunflower seeds and pepper as needed
- ½ cup pistachios, finely chopped
- Juice of 1 lemon
- 1 teaspoon extra virgin olive oil

How To

1. Preheat your oven to 350 degrees F.

2. Line a baking sheet with parchment paper and keep it on the side.

3. Pat fish dry with kitchen towels and lightly season with sunflower seeds and pepper.

4. Take a small bowl and stir in pistachios.

5. Place the sole on the prepped sheet and press 2 tablespoons of pistachio mixture on top of each fillet.

6. Drizzle fish with lemon juice and olive oil.

7. Bake for 10 minutes until the top is golden and fish flakes with a fork.

8. Serve and enjoy!

Nutrition Values (Per Serving)

- Calories: 166
- Fat: 6g
- Carbohydrates: 2g
- Protein: 26g

Cajun Jambalaya Soup

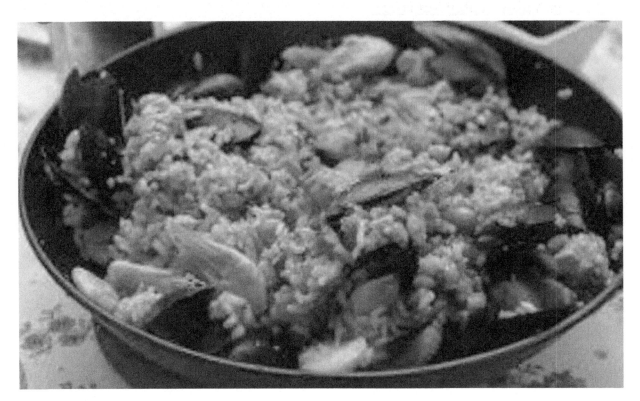

Serving: 6

Prep Time: 15 minutes

Cook Time: 40 minutes

Ingredients

- 1-pound large shrimp, raw and deveined
- 4 ounces chicken, diced
- ¼ cup Frank's red-hot sauce
- 2 cups okra
- 3 tablespoons Cajun seasoning
- 2 bay leaves
- ½ head cauliflower
- 1 large can organic, diced
- 1 large onion, chopped
- 2 cloves garlic, diced
- 5 cups chicken stock
- 4 pepper

How To

1. Take a heavy-bottomed pot and add all ingredients except cauliflower.

2. Place it over on high heat.
3. Mix them well and bring it to boil.
4. Once boiled, lower the heat to simmer.
5. Simmer for 30 minutes.
6. Rice the cauliflower in your blender.
7. Stir into the pot and simmer for another 5 minutes.
8. Serve and enjoy!

Nutrition Values (Per Serving)

- Calories: 143
- Fat: 3g
- Carbohydrates: 14g
- Protein: 18g

Anti-Inflammatory Turmeric Gummies

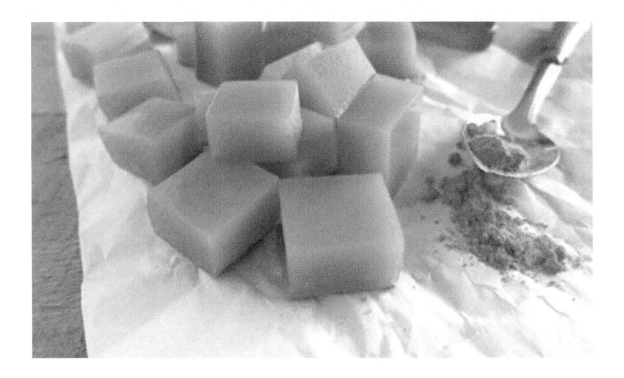

Serving: 6

Prep Time: 4 hours

Cook Time: 10 minutes

Ingredients

- 1 teaspoon turmeric, grounded
- 8 tablespoons gelatin powder, unflavored
- 6 tablespoons maple syrup
- 3 ½ cups of water

How To

1. Take a pot and combine maple syrup, turmeric, and water.
2. Bring it to boil for 5 minutes.
3. Remove from the heat and sprinkle with gelatin powder.
4. Mix to hydrate the gelatin.
5. Then turn on the heat again and bring to a boil till the gelatin dissolves properly.
6. Take a dish and pour the mixture.
7. Let it chill for 4 hours in your refrigerator.
8. Once ready, slice and serve.
9. Enjoy!

Nutrition Values (Per Serving)

- Calories: 68
- Fat: 0.03g
- Carbohydrates: 17g
- Protein: 0.2g

Delicious Snow Crab

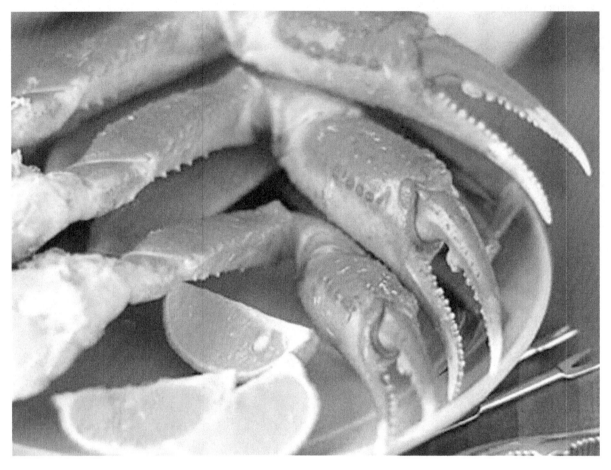

Serving: 2

Prep Time: 10 minutes

Cook Time: 10 minutes

Ingredients

- 1 lemon, fresh and quartered
- 3 tablespoons Cajun seasoning
- 2 bay leaves
- 4 snow crab legs, precooked and defrosted
- Golden ghee

How To

1. Take a large pot and fill it about halfway with salted water.
2. Bring the water to a boil.
3. Squeeze lemon juice into a pot and toss in remaining lemon quarters.
4. Add bay leaves and Cajun seasoning.

5. Then season for 1 minute.

6. Add crab legs and boil for 8 minutes (make sure to keep them submerged the whole time).

7. Melt ghee in microwave and use as a dipping sauce, enjoy!

Nutrition (Per Serving)

- Calories: 643
- Fat: 51g
- Carbohydrates: 3g
- Protein: 41g

Blackberry Chicken Wings

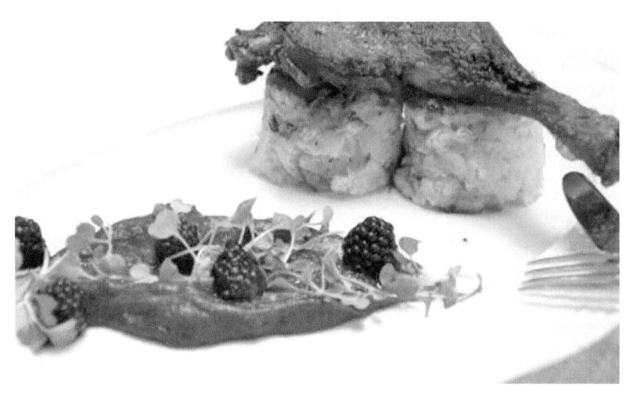

Serving: 4

Prep Time: 35 minutes

Cook Time: 50minutes

Ingredients

- 3 pounds chicken wings, about 20 pieces
- ½ cup blackberry chipotle jam
- Sunflower seeds and pepper to taste
- ½ cup of water

How To

1. Add water and jam to a bowl and mix well.
2. Place chicken wings in a zip bag and add two-thirds of marinade.
3. Season with sunflower seeds and pepper.
4. Let it marinate for 30 minutes.
5. Preheat your oven to 400-degree F.
6. Prepare a baking sheet and wire rack, place chicken wings in a wire rack and bake for 15 minutes.
7. Brush remaining marinade and bake for 30 minutes more.
8. Enjoy!

Nutrition Values (Per Serving)

- Calories: 502
- Fat: 39g
- Carbohydrates: 01.8g
- Protein: 34g

Shredded Cabbage and Rotisserie Chicken

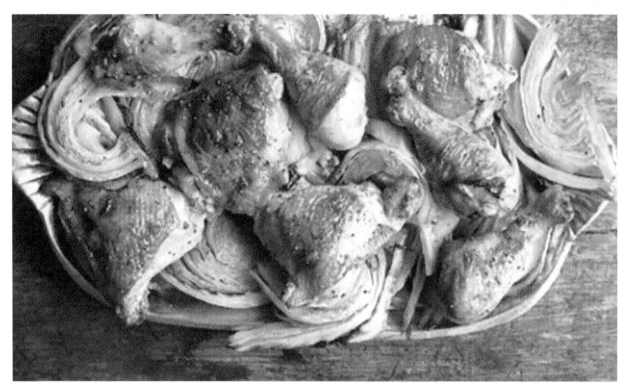

Serving: 4

Prep Time: 5 minutes

Cook Time: Nil

Ingredients

- 1 pound rotisserie chicken, cooked
- 7 ounces fresh green cabbage
- ½ red onion
- 1 tablespoon olive oil
- ½ cup mayonnaise, homemade
- Salt and pepper to taste

How To

1. Shred the cabbage using a sharp knife and transfer to a plate.
2. Slice the onion thinly and add them to the plate.
3. Add rotisserie chicken to a plate and add mayo.
4. Drizzle olive oil.
5. Season accordingly and toss.
6. Serve!

Nutrition (Per Serving)

- Calories: 423
- Fat: 35g
- Carbohydrates: 6g
- Protein: 17g

Lemon and Butter Cod

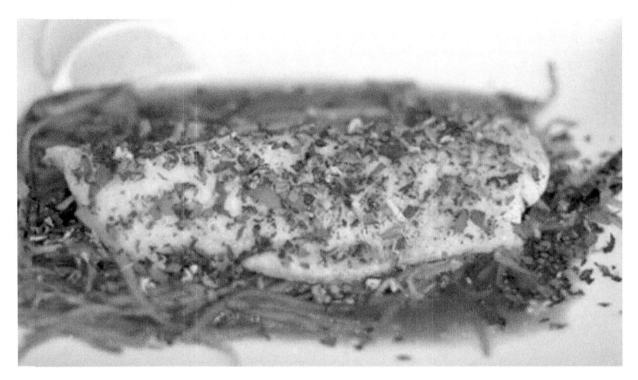

Serving: 3

Prep Time: 5 minutes

Cook Time: 20 minutes

Ingredients

- 4 tablespoons salted almond butter, divided
- 4 thyme sprigs, fresh and divided
- 4 teaspoons lemon juice, fresh and divided
- 4 cod fillets, 6 ounces each
- Salt to taste

How To

1. Preheat your oven to 400 degrees F.
2. Season cod fillets with salt on both side.
3. Take four pieces of foil; each foil should be three times bigger than the fillets.
4. Divide fillets between the foils and top with butter, lemon juice, thyme.
5. Fold to form a pouch and transfer pouches to a baking sheet.
6. Bake for 20 minutes.
7. Open and let the steam out.
8. Serve and enjoy!

Nutrition (Per Serving)

- Calories: 284
- Fat: 18g
- Carbohydrates: 1g
- Protein: 32g

Chapter 6: Snack Recipes

Coconut Cookies

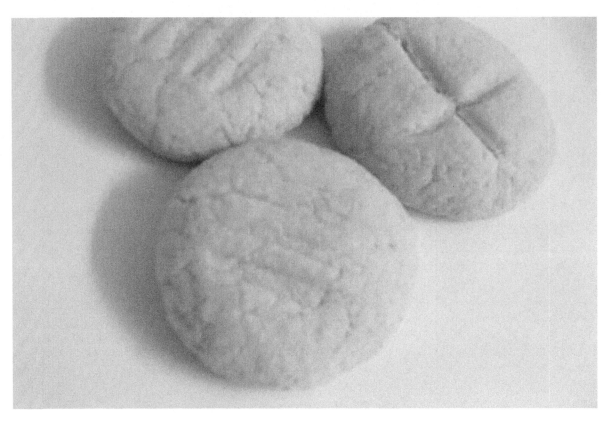

Serving: 10-15

Prep Time: 10 minutes

Cook Time: 0 minutes

Ingredients

- ¾ cup of coconut flour
- 2 cups of smooth cashew butter
- ½ cup of pure maple syrup
- 1-2 tablespoon of sprinkles

How To

1. Take a large-sized baking tray and line it with parchment paper.
2. Take a large-sized mixing bowl and add coconut flour.
3. Add the cashew butter and maple syrup and mix the whole mixture until it is nice and combined.
4. Stir the sprinkles.

5. Add some more coconut flour if the batter is too thin.
6. Alternatively, add some water if the batter is too thick.
7. Form small balls using the batter and place them on your parchment paper.
8. Press the balls into a cookie shape.
9. Allow them to chill for a while and serve!

Nutrition Values (Per Serving)

- Calories: 110
- Fat: 2g
- Carbohydrates: 4g
- Protein: 18g

Bean Balls

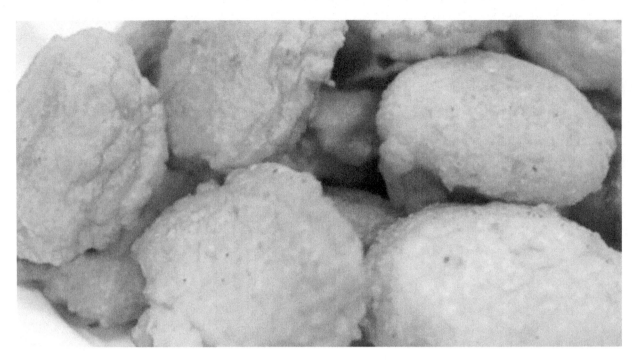

Serving: 30

Prep Time: 10 minutes

Cook Time: 0 minutes

Ingredients

- ½ cup of dates
- ½ cup of dried berries and cherries
- ½ cup of ground almonds
- 2 tablespoons of cocoa
- 2 tablespoons of runny Agave Nectar
- 3 ¾ cups of Black beans
- 1 small orange zest

As for topping

- Cocoa
- Coconut
- Toasted Pistachios

How To

1. Take a food processor and add dates, ground almonds, cocoa, honey, cherries, black beans, orange zest.
2. Process the food well until they are finely chopped up.

3. Use your hand to roll up the mixture into balls.
4. Garnish the balls with toasted cocoa, pistachios, or coconut.
5. Serve or store in the fridge.

Nutrition Values (Per Serving)

- Calories: 366
- Fat: 14g
- Carbohydrates: 96g
- Protein: 8g

Delicious Eggplant Salad

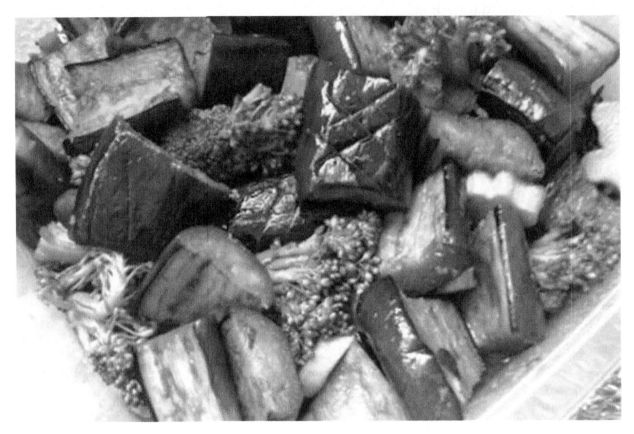

Serving: 3

Prep Time: 10 minutes

Cook Time: 30 minutes

Ingredients

- 2 eggplants, peeled and sliced
- 2 garlic cloves
- 2 green bell peppers, sliced, seeds removed
- ½ cup fresh parsley
- ½ cup mayonnaise, homemade
- Salt and black pepper

How To

1. Preheat your oven to 480 degrees F.
2. Take a baking pan and add eggplants and black pepper to it.
3. Bake for about 30 minutes.
4. Flip the vegetables after 20 minutes.
5. Then, take a bowl and add baked vegetables and all the remaining ingredients.

6. Mix it well.

7. Serve and enjoy!

Nutrition (Per Serving)

- Calories: 196
- Fat: 108.g
- Carbohydrates: 13.4g
- Protein: 14.6g

Simple Cabbage Slaw

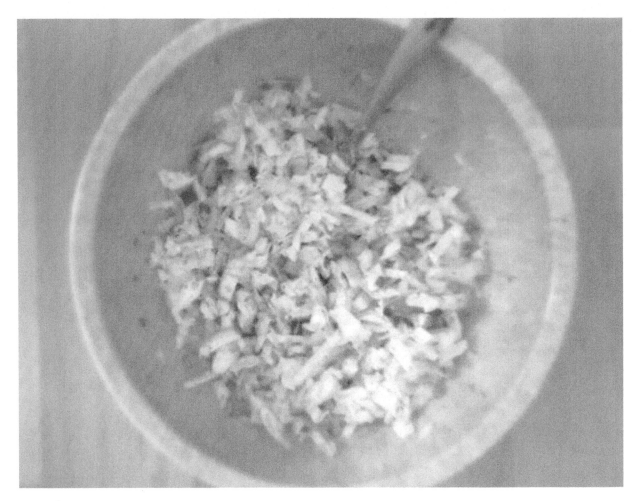

Serving: 6

Prep Time: 10 minutes

Cook Time: Nil

Ingredients

- 12 ounces green and red cabbage, shredded and mixed
- 4 ounces kale, chopped
- 1 cup Keto-Friendly mayonnaise, homemade
- ½ teaspoon each salt and pepper

How To

1. Add listed ingredients to a bowl and mix well using a spatula.
2. Serve immediately or chilled.
3. Enjoy!

Nutrition (Per Serving)

- Calories: 266
- Fat: 26g
- Carbohydrates: 6g
- Protein: 0.6g

Creative Lemon and Broccoli Dish

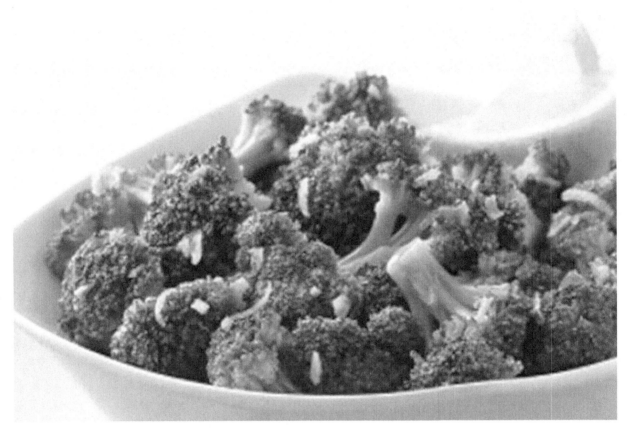

Serving: 6

Prep Time: 10 minutes

Cook Time: 15 minutes

Ingredients

- 2 heads broccoli, separated into florets
- 2 teaspoons extra virgin olive oil
- 1 teaspoon salt
- ½ teaspoon black pepper
- 1 garlic clove, minced
- ½ teaspoon lemon juice

How To

1. Preheat your oven to 400 degrees F.
2. Take a large-sized bowl and add broccoli florets.
3. Drizzle olive oil and season with pepper, salt, and garlic.
4. Spread the broccoli out in a single even layer on a baking sheet.
5. Bake for 15-20 minutes until fork tender.

6. Squeeze lemon juice on top.

7. Serve and enjoy!

Nutrition (Per Serving)

- Calories: 49
- Fat: 1.9g
- Carbohydrates: 7g
- Protein: 3g

Seemingly Easy Portobello Mushrooms

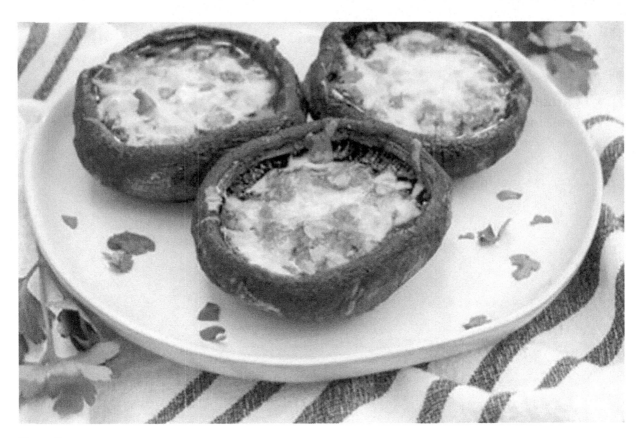

Serving: 4

Prep Time: 10 minutes

Cook Time: 10 minutes

Ingredients

- 12 cherry tomatoes
- 2 ounces scallions
- 4 portabella mushrooms
- 4 ¼ ounces of almond butter
- Salt and pepper to taste

How To

1. Take a large skillet and melt the butter over medium heat.
2. Add mushrooms and sauté for 3 minutes.
3. Stir in cherry tomatoes and scallions.
4. Sauté for 5 minutes.
5. Season accordingly.
6. Sauté until veggies are tender.

7. Enjoy!

<u>Nutrition (Per Serving)</u>

- Calories: 154
- Fat: 10g
- Carbohydrates: 2g
- Protein: 7g

Almond Breaded Crunchy Chicken Bread

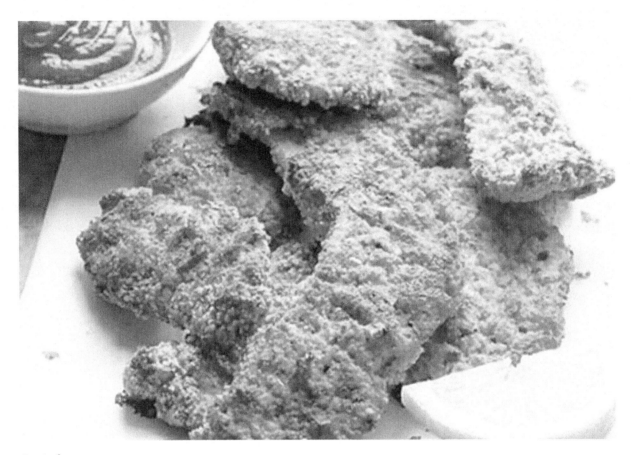

Serving: 3

Prep Time: 15 minutes

Cook Time: 15 minutes

Ingredients

- 2 large chicken breasts, boneless and skinless
- 1/3 cup lemon juice
- 1 ½ cups seasoned almond meal
- 2 tablespoons coconut oil
- Lemon pepper, to taste
- Parsley for decoration

How To

1. Slice chicken breast in half.
2. Pound out each half until ¼ inch thick.
3. Take a pan and place it over medium heat, add oil and heat it up.
4. Dip each chicken breast slice into lemon juice and let it sit for 2 minutes.

5. Turnover and let the other side sit for 2 minutes as well.

6. Transfer to almond meal and coat both sides.

7. Add coated chicken to the oil and fry for 4 minutes per side, making sure to sprinkle lemon pepper liberally.

8. Transfer to a paper-lined sheet and repeat until all chicken is fried.

9. Garnish with parsley and enjoy!

Nutrition Values (Per Serving)

- Calories: 325
- Fat: 24g
- Carbohydrates: 3g
- Protein: 16g

Yogurt and Cucumber Salad

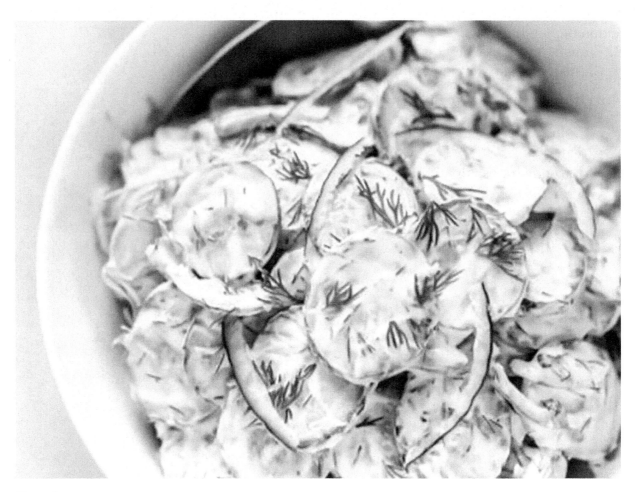

Serving: 4

Prep Time: 10 minutes

Cook Time: Nil

Ingredients

- 5-6 small cucumbers, peeled and diced
- 1 (8 ounces) container plain Greek yogurt
- 2 garlic cloves, minced
- 1 tablespoon fresh mint, minced
- Sea sunflower seeds and fresh black pepper

How To

1. Take a large bowl and add cucumbers, garlic, yogurt, mint.

2. Season with sunflower seeds and pepper.

3. Refrigerate the salad for 1 hour and serve.

4. Enjoy!

Nutrition Values (Per Serving)

- Calories: 74
- Fat: 0.7g
- Carbohydrates: 16g
- Protein: 2g

Chicken Breast Salad

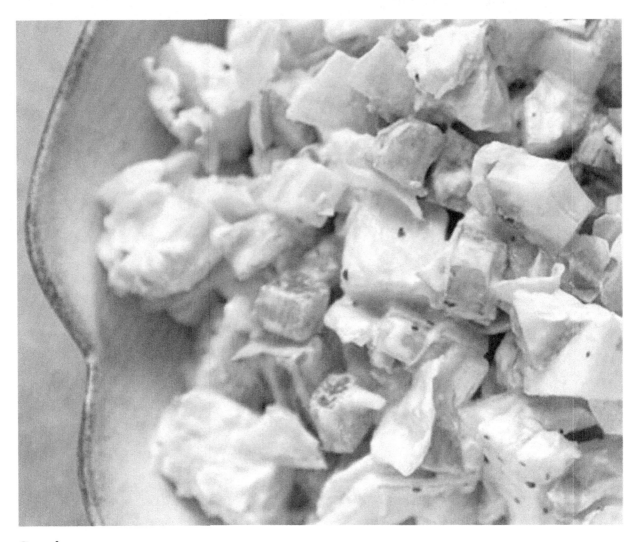

Serving: 4

Prep Time: 25 minutes

Cook Time: 30-55 minutes

Ingredients

- 3 ½ ounces chicken breast
- 2 tablespoons spinach
- 1 ¾ ounces lettuces
- 1 bell pepper
- 2 tablespoons olive oil
- Lemon juice to taste

How To

1. Boil the chicken breast without adding salt, cut the meat into small strips.
2. Put the spinach in boiling water for a few minutes, cut into small strips.
3. Cut pepper in strips as well.
4. Add everything to a bowl and mix with juice and oil.
5. Serve!

Nutrition Values (Per Serving)

- Calories: 100
- Fat: 11g
- Carbohydrates: 3g
- Protein: 6g

Red Pepper Roast and Hummus

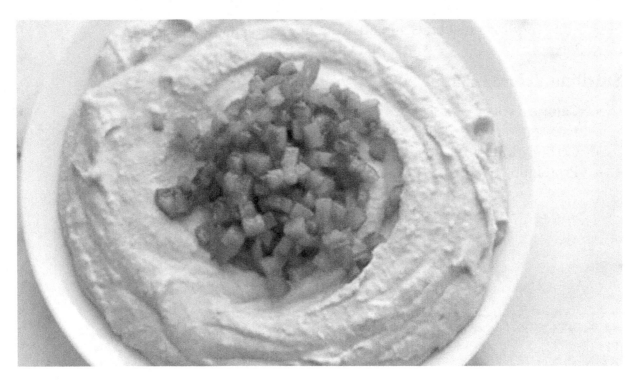

Serving: 4

Prep Time: 5 minutes

Cook Time: 0 minute

Ingredients

- 1 cup chickpea, cooked
- 2 whole red pepper, roasted, seeded, and peeled
- 4 tablespoons lemon juice
- 3 tablespoons olive oil
- 2 teaspoons garlic, minced
- 1 teaspoon salt
- 1 teaspoon black pepper

How To

1. Add all ingredients to your blender.
2. Pulse until you get a smooth mixture.
3. Serve with chips and enjoy!

Nutrition Values (Per Serving)
- Calories: 293
- Fat: 12g

- Carbohydrates: 35g
- Protein: 11g

Spiced Up Crunchy Taro

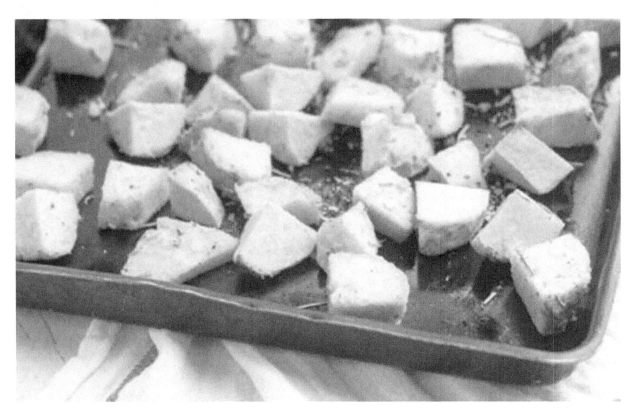

Serving: 2

Prep Time: 10 minutes

Cook Time: 20 minutes

Ingredients

- 2 cups taro, sliced thinly
- 1 tablespoon olive oil
- 1 teaspoon cayenne pepper powder
- A pinch salt

How To

1. Preheat your oven to 350 degrees F.
2. Take a bowl and combine all ingredients.
3. Toss to coat the taro with the spices and seasoning.
4. Place the taro slices on a baking rack.
5. Bake for 20 minutes.
6. Serve and enjoy!

Nutrition Values (Per Serving)

- Calories: 176
- Fat: 1g
- Carbohydrates: 28g
- Protein: 2g

Orange and Onion Salad

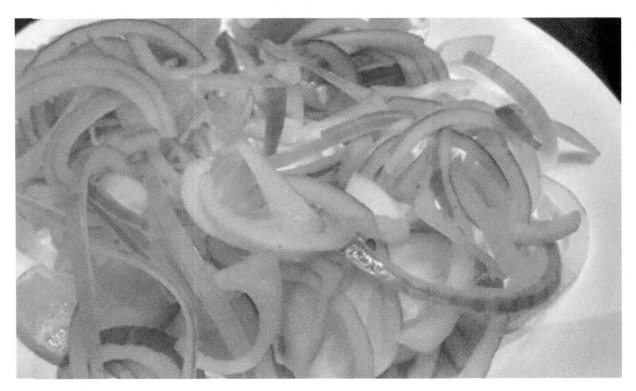

Serving: 3

Prep Time: 10 minutes

Cook Time: nil

Ingredients

- 6 large oranges
- 3 tablespoons of red wine vinegar
- 6 tablespoons of olive oil
- 1 teaspoon of dried oregano
- 1 red onion, thinly sliced
- 1 cup olive oil
- ¼ cup of fresh chives, chopped
- Ground black pepper

How To

1. Peel the orange and cut each of them into 4-5 crosswise slices.
2. Transfer the oranges to a shallow dish.
3. Drizzle vinegar, olive oil and sprinkle oregano.
4. Toss.
5. Chill for 30 minutes.

6. Arrange sliced onion and black olives on top.

7. Decorate with an additional sprinkle of chives and a fresh grind of pepper.

8. Serve and enjoy!

Nutrition Values (Per Serving)

- Calories: 120
- Fat: 6g
- Carbohydrates: 20g
- Protein: 2g

Proper Sauteed Green Beans

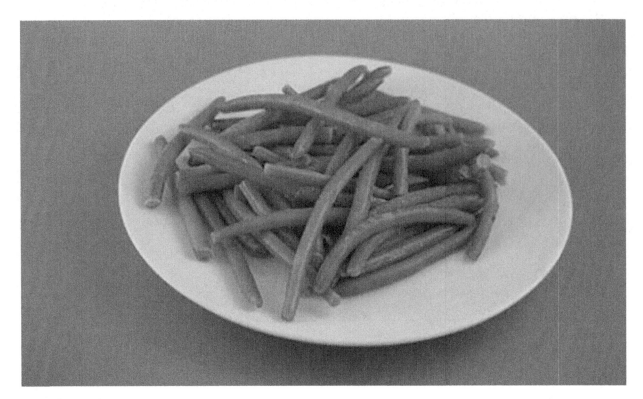

Serving: 6

Prep Time: 5 minutes

Cook Time: 6 minutes

Ingredients

- 3 pounds green beans, ends trimmed
- 3 tablespoons olive oil
- 3 shallots, chopped
- 4 clove garlic, minced
- Salt and pepper, to taste

How To

1. Take a skillet and add oil.
2. Heat the oil over medium heat.
3. Sauté the garlic and shallots until fragrant.
4. Add in the green beans.
5. Season with salt and pepper to taste.
6. Keep sautéing for 5 minutes.
7. Serve and enjoy!

<u>Nutrition Values (Per Serving)</u>

- Calories: 116
- Fat: 8g
- Carbohydrates: 11g
- Protein: 3g

Medi-Peanut Butter Popcorn

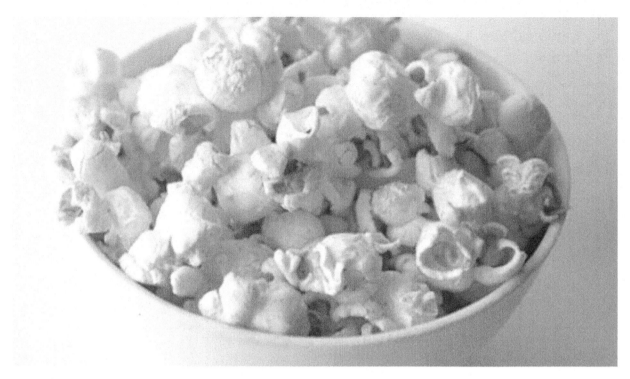

Serving: 4

Prep Time: 5 minutes + 20 minutes chill time

Cook Time: 2-3 minutes

Ingredients

- 3 cups Medjool dates, chopped
- 12 ounces brewed coffee
- 1 cup pecan, chopped
- ½ cup coconut, shredded
- ½ cup of cocoa powder

How To

1. Soak dates in warm coffee for 5 minutes.
2. Remove dates from coffee and mash them, making a fine smooth mixture.
3. Stir in remaining ingredients (except cocoa powder) and form small balls out of the mixture.
4. Coat with cocoa powder, serve and enjoy!

Nutrition(Per Serving)

- Calories: 265
- Fat: 12g

- Carbohydrates: 43g
- Protein 3g

Zesty Oven Baked Sweet Potatoes

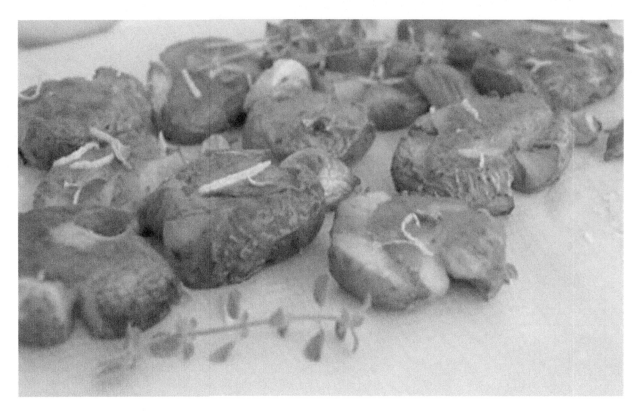

Prep Time: 10 minutes

Cook Time: 30 minute

Serving: 7

Ingredients

- ¼ teaspoon of pepper
- Vegetable cooking spray
- 1 tablespoon parsley, chopped
- 1 teaspoon orange, rind
- 1 garlic clove, minced

Process

1. Take a large-sized bowl and add the first 4 ingredients.
2. Toss everything well.
3. Take a large baking sheet and grease it with cooking spray.
4. Arrange your sweet potato slices in a single layer.
5. Preheat your oven to a temperature of 400 degrees F and let it cook for about 30 minutes.
6. Make sure to turn the potatoes after 15 minutes.
7. Take a small bowl and add parsley, garlic, and orange rind.

8. Mix them well.

9. Sprinkle the parsley all over the baked potato slices and serve!

Nutrition Values (Per Serving

- Calories: 178
- Fat: 25g
- Carbohydrates: 366g
- Protein: 25g

Roasted Plums

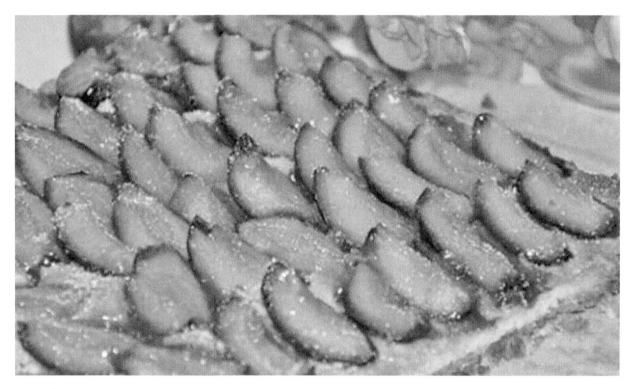

Serving: 3

Prep Time: 10 minutes

Cook Time: 15 minutes

- 4 pieces of plums, pitted and halved
- ½ cup of orange juice
- 2 tablespoons of packed brown sugar
- ½ teaspoon of cinnamon, ground
- 1/8 teaspoon of nutmeg, ground
- 1/8 teaspoon of cumin
- 1/8 teaspoon of cardamom
- ¼ cup of toasted and slivered almonds

Cook Directions

1. Preheat your oven to 400-degree F.
2. Take a shallow baking dish and grease it with cooking spray.
3. Add your plums to the pan with the cut side facing up.
4. Take a bowl and whisk in orange juice, cinnamon, brown sugar, cumin, nutmeg, and cardamom.

5. Drizzle the mixture over your plums.

6. Bake for 20 minutes until the plums are hot and the sauce shows a bubbly texture.

7. Top with some almonds and enjoy!

Nutrition Values (Per Serving)

- Calories: 113
- Fats: 4g
- Carbs: 20g
- Protein: 2.1g

Guilty and Dairy Free Pudding

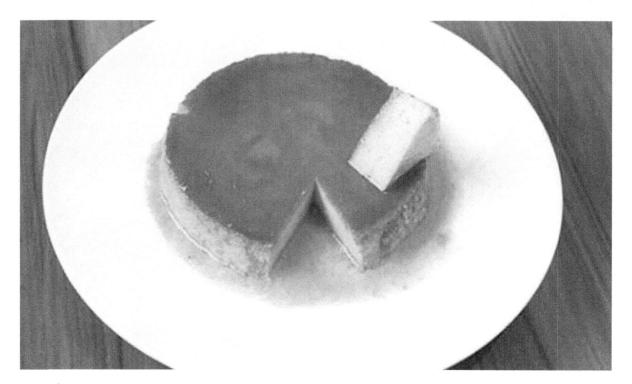

Serving: 4

Prep Time: 10 minutes

Cook Time: 10 minutes

Ingredients

- 3 tablespoons of cornstarch
- 2 tablespoons of water
- 1 ½ cups of soy milk
- ¼ teaspoon of vanilla extract
- ¼ cup of white sugar
- ¼ cup of unsweetened cocoa powder

Cook Directions

1. Take a small-sized bowl, add cornstarch and water and mix well to form a nice paste-like texture.

2. Take a large-sized saucepan and place it over medium heat.

3. Add soy milk, sugar, vanilla, cocoa, and your prepared cornstarch mixture.

4. Give the whole mixture a stir and allow it to cook until boiling point is reached.

5. Keep stirring until the mixture is thick.

6. Remove the heat.

7. Allow it to cool and chill in your fridge until it is fully cooled and has settled in.

8. Enjoy!

Nutrition Values (Per Serving)

- Calories: 267
- Fats: 5g
- Carbs:53g
- Protein:8g

Crunchy Flax and Almond Crackers

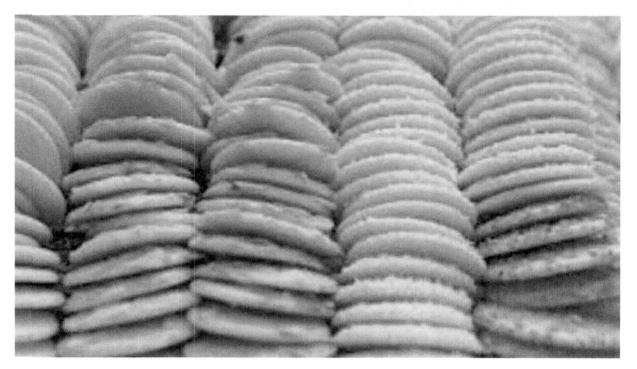

Serving: 20-24 crackers

Prep Time: 15 minutes

Cooking Time: 60 minutes

Ingredients:

- ½ cup ground flax seeds
- ½ cup almond flour
- 1 tablespoon coconut flour
- 2 tablespoons shelled hemp seeds
- ¼ teaspoon sunflower seeds
- 1 egg white
- 2 tablespoons unsalted almond butter, melted

How To:

1. Preheat your oven to 300 degrees F.
2. Line a baking sheet with parchment paper, keep it on the side.
3. Add flax, almond, coconut flour, hemp seed, seeds to a bowl and mix.
4. Add egg and melted almond butter, mix until combined.
5. Transfer dough to a sheet of parchment paper and cover with another sheet of paper.
6. Roll out dough.
7. Cut into crackers and bake for 60 minutes.
8. Let them cool and enjoy!

Nutrition Values (Per Serving)

- Total Carbs: 1.2 (%)
- Fiber: 1g
- Protein: 2g (%)
- Fat: 6g (%)

Ginger Date Bars

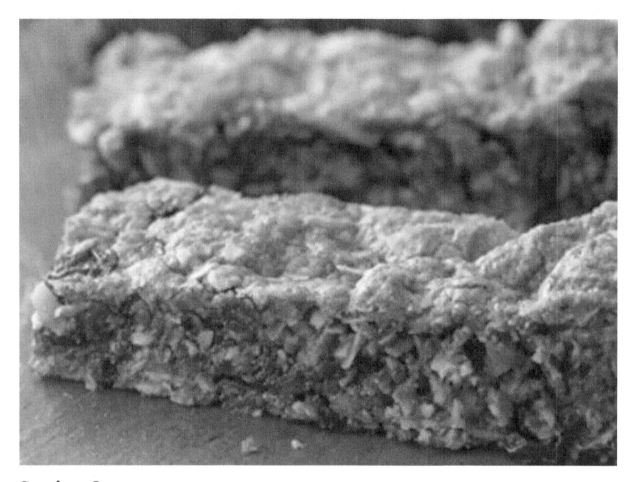

Serving: 8

Prep Time: 10 minutes

Cook Time: 20 minutes

Ingredients

- ¾ cup dates pitted
- 1 ½ cups almond, soaked in overnight water
- ¼ cup almond milk
- 1 teaspoon ginger, grounded

How To

1. Preheat your oven to 350 degrees F.
2. Place the almond in a food processor.
3. Pulse it until you get a thick dough form.
4. Press the dough in a baking dish lined with parchment paper.
5. Set it aside.

6. Make a date mix by combining the rest of the ingredients in your food processor.
7. Pour the date mixture on to the almond crust.
8. Bake for 20 minutes.
9. Allow it to cool before you slice them.
10. Serve and enjoy!

Nutrition Values (Per Serving)

- Calories: 45
- Fat: 0.3g
- Carbohydrates: 11g
- Protein: 0.5g

Zingy Onion and Thyme Crackers

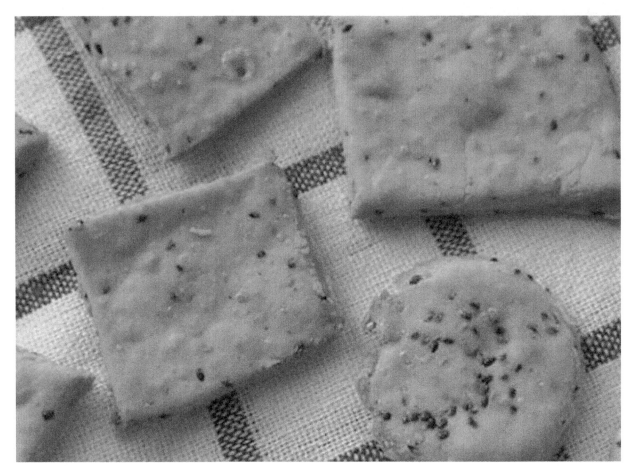

Serving: 75 crackers

Prep Time: 15 minutes

Cooking Time: 120 minutes

Ingredients:

- 1 garlic clove, minced
- 1 cup sweet onion, coarsely chopped
- 2 teaspoons fresh thyme leaves
- ¼ cup avocado oil
- ¼ teaspoon garlic powder
- Freshly ground black pepper
- ¼ cup sunflower seeds
- 1 ½ cups roughly ground flax seeds

How To:

1. Preheat your oven to 225 degrees F.

2. Line two baking sheets with parchment paper and keep it on the side.
3. Add garlic, onion, thyme, oil, sunflower seeds, and pepper to a food processor.
4. Add sunflower and flax seeds, pulse until pureed.
5. Transfer batter to prepared baking sheets and spread evenly, cut into crackers
6. Bake for 60 minutes.
7. Remove parchment paper and flip crackers, bake for another hour.
8. If crackers are thick, it will take more time.
9. Remove from oven and let them cool.
10. Enjoy!

Nutritional Contents:

- Total Carbs: 0.8g (%)
- Fiber: 0.2g
- Protein: 0.4g (%)
- Fat: 2.7g (%)

Chapter 7: Dinner Recipes
Spicy Paprika Lamb Chops

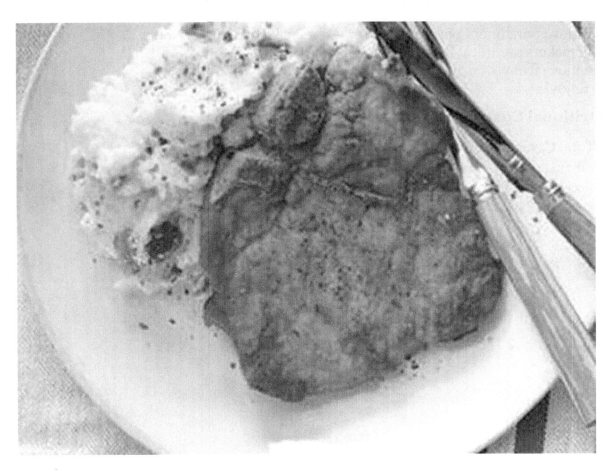

Serving: 4

Prep Time: 10 minutes

Cook Time: 15 minutes

Ingredients

- 1 lamb rack, cut into chops
- Pepper to taste
- 1 tablespoon paprika
- 1/2 cup cumin powder
- 1/2 teaspoon chili powder

How To

1. Take a bowl and add paprika, cumin, chili, pepper, and stir.

2. Add lamb chops and rub the mixture.

3. Heat grill over medium-temperature and add lamb chops, cook for 5 minutes.

4. Flip and cook for 5 minutes more; flip again.

5. Cook for 2 minutes, flip and cook for 2 minutes more.

6. Serve and enjoy!

<u>Nutrition Values (Per Serving)</u>

- Calories: 200
- Fat: 5g
- Carbohydrates: 4g
- Protein: 8g

Original Japanese Croquettes

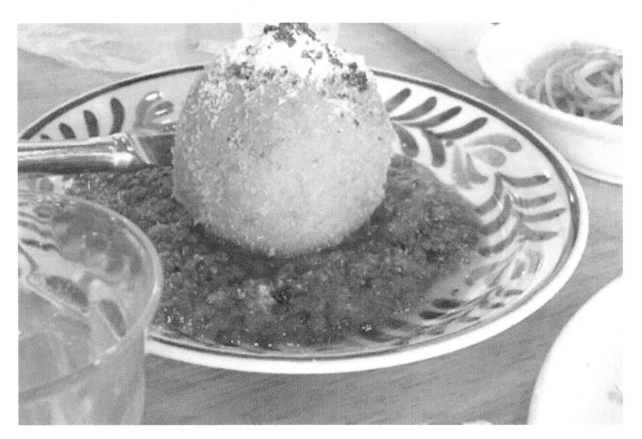

Serving: 10

Prep Time: 10 minute

Cook Time: 20 minutes

Ingredients

- 3 medium russet potatoes. Peeled and chopped
- 1 tablespoon butter
- 1 tablespoon vegetable oil
- 3 onions, diced
- ¾ pound ground beef
- All-purpose flour for coating
- 2 eggs, beaten
- Panko bread crumbs for coating
- ½ cup oil, frying

Directions

1. Take a saucepan and place it over medium-high heat, add potatoes and salted water, boil for 16 minutes.

2. Remove water and put potatoes in another bowl, add butter and mash the potatoes.

3. Take a frying pan and place it over medium heat, add 1 tablespoon oil and let it heat up.

4. Add onions and stir fry until tender.

5. Keep frying until beef is browned.

6. Mix in beef with potatoes evenly.

7. Take another frying pan and place it over medium heat; add half a cup of oil.

8. Form croquettes using the mashed potato mixture and coat them with flour, then eggs, and finally, breadcrumbs.

9. Fry patties until golden on all sides.

10. Enjoy!

Nutrition Values (Per Serving)

- Calories: 239
- Fat: 4g
- Carbohydrates: 20g
- Protein: 10g

Perfect Eggplant Salad

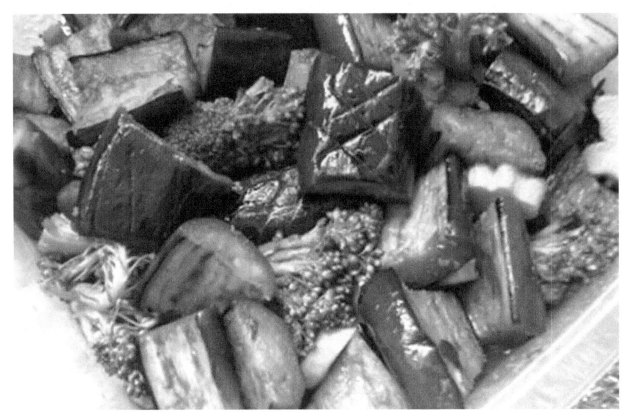

Serving: 8

Prep Time: 20 minutes

Cook Time: 15 minutes

Ingredients

- 1 large eggplant, washed and cubed
- 1 tomato, seeded and chopped
- 1 small onion, diced
- 2 tablespoons extra virgin olive oil
- ½ cup feta cheese, crumbled

How To

1. Preheat your outdoor grill to medium-high.
2. Pierce the eggplant a few times using a knife/fork.
3. Cook the eggplants on your grill for about 15 minutes until they are charred.
4. Keep it on the side and allow them to cool.
5. Remove the skin from the eggplant and dice the pulp.
6. Transfer the pulp to mixing bowl and add onion, tomato, olive oil, feta cheese.
7. Mix well and chill for 1 hour.

8. Season with salt and enjoy!

Nutrition (Per Serving)

- Calories: 99
- Fat: 7g
- Carbohydrates: 7g
- Protein:3.4g

Pistachio and Brussels

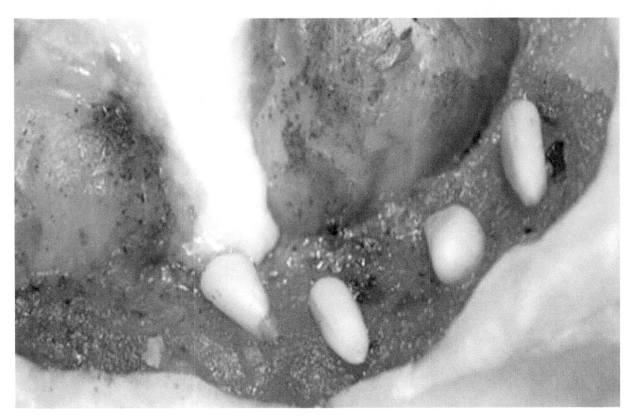

Serving: 4

Prep Time: 15 minutes

Cook Time: 15 minutes

Ingredients

- 1 pound Brussels sprouts, tough bottom trimmed and halved lengthwise
- 1 tablespoon extra-virgin olive oil
- Salt and pepper as needed
- ½ cup roasted pistachios, chopped
- Juice of ½ lemon

How To

1. Preheat your oven to 400 degrees F.
2. Line a baking sheet with aluminum foil and keep it on the side.
3. Take a large bowl and add Brussels sprouts with olive oil and coat well.
4. Season sea salt, pepper, spread veggies evenly on the sheet.
5. Bake for 15 minutes until lightly caramelized.
6. Remove the oven and transfer to a serving bowl.
7. Toss with pistachios and lemon juice.

8. Serve warm and enjoy!

Nutrition (Per Serving)

- Calories: 126
- Fat: 7g
- Carbohydrates: 14g
- Protein: 6g

Warm Medi Tilapia

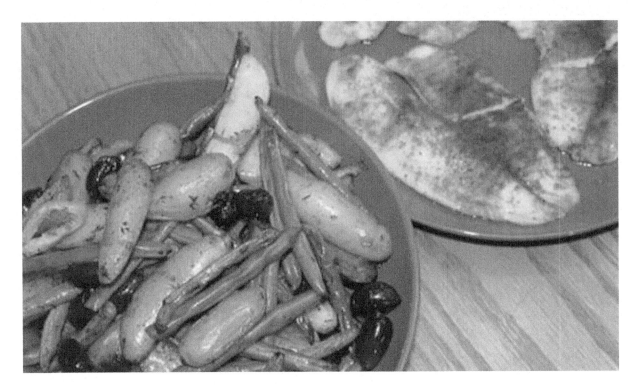

Serving: 4

Prep Time: 15 minutes

Cook Time: 15 minute

Ingredients

- 3 tablespoons sun-dried tomatoes, packed in oil, drained and chopped
- 1 tablespoon capers, drained
- 2 tilapia fillets
- 1 tablespoon oil from sun-dried tomatoes
- 2 tablespoons kalamata olives, chopped and pitted

How To

1. Preheat your oven to 372 degrees F.
2. Take a small-sized bowl and add sun-dried tomatoes, olives, capers and stir well.
3. Keep the mixture on the side.
4. Take a baking sheet and transfer the tilapia fillets and arrange them side by side.
5. Drizzle olive oil all over them.
6. Bake in your oven for 10-15 minutes.
7. After 10 minutes, check the fish for a "Flaky" texture.
8. Once cooked properly, top the fish with tomato mixture and serve!

Nutrition (Per Serving)

- Calories: 183
- Fat: 8g
- Carbohydrates: 18g
- Protein:83g

Garlic Dredged Green Beans

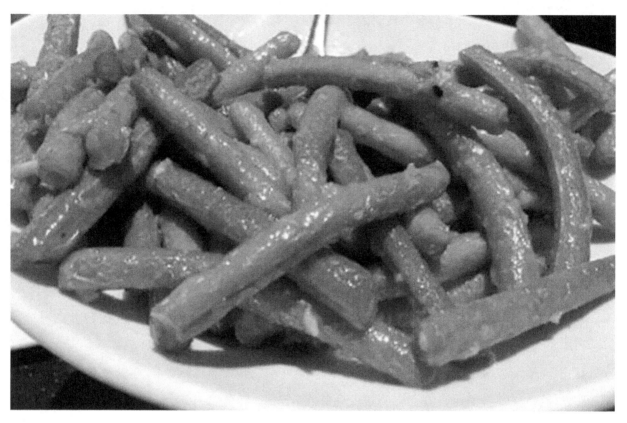

Serving: 4

Prep Time: 5 minutes

Cook Time: 20 minutes

Ingredients

- 1 bunch of leafy greens

Sauce

- ½ cup of cashews soaked in water for 10 minutes
- ¼ cup of water
- 1 tablespoon of lemon juice
- 1 teaspoon of coconut aminos
- 1 clove peeled the whole clove
- 1/8 teaspoon of flavored vinegar

How To

1. Make the sauce by draining and discard the soaking water from your cashews and add the cashews to a blender.
2. Add fresh water, lemon juice, flavored vinegar, coconut aminos, garlic.
3. Blitz until you have a smooth cream and transfer to a bowl.
4. Add ½ cup of water to the pot.
5. Place the steamer basket into the pot and add the greens to the basket.
6. Lock up the lid and steam for 1 minute.
7. Quick-release the pressure.
8. Transfer the steamed greens to a strainer and extract excess water.
9. Place the greens into a mixing bowl.
10. Add lemon garlic sauce and toss.
11. Enjoy!

Nutrition Values (Per Serving)

- Calories: 77
- Fat: 5g
- Carbohydrates: 0g
- Protein: 2g

Simple Baked Chicken

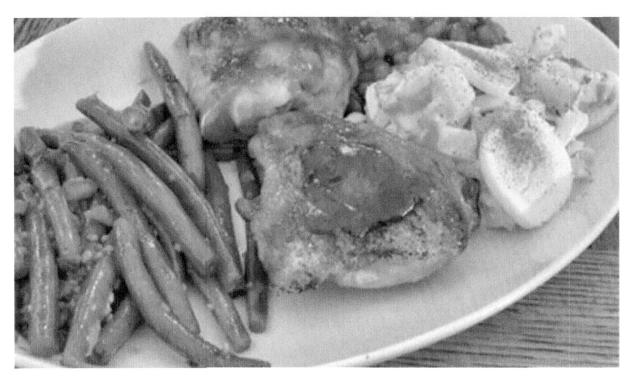

Serving: 2

Prep Time: 10 minutes

Cook Time: 40 minutes

Ingredients

- 2 pieces of 8 ounces skinless and boneless chicken breast
- Salt and pepper as needed
- ¼ cup of olive oil and lemon juice (equal amount)
- ½ teaspoon of dried oregano
- ¼ teaspoon of dried thyme

How To

1. Season breast by rubbing salt and pepper on all sides.
2. Transfer the chicken to a bowl.
3. Take another bowl and add olive oil, oregano, lemon juice, thyme and mix well.
4. Pour the prepared marinade over the chicken breast and allow it to marinate for 10 minutes.
5. Preheat your oven to 400 degrees F.
6. Set the oven rack about 6 inches above the heat source.
7. Transfer the chicken breast to a baking sheet and pour extra marinade on top.
8. Bake for 35-45 minutes until the center is no longer pink.

9. Remove it and place it on the top rack.
10.   Broil for 5 minutes more.
11. Enjoy and serve!

Nutrition(Per Serving)

- Calories: 501
- Fat: 32g
- Carbohydrates: 3.5g
- Protein: 47g

Hearty Halibut

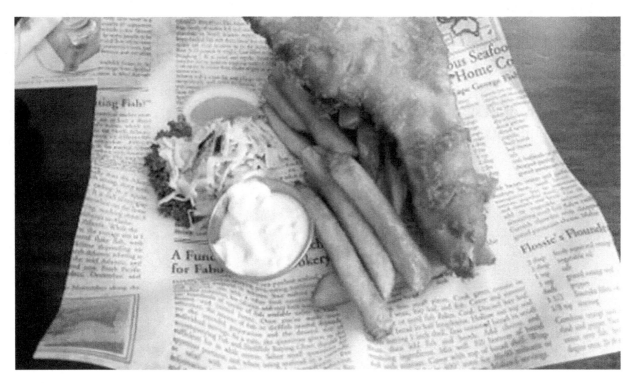

Serving: 6

Prep Time: 5 minutes

Cook Time: 20 minutes

Ingredients

- 2 pounds halibut fillets
- 2 stalks celery, chopped
- 4 cloves garlic, minced
- 2 tablespoons olive oil
- 1/2 cup parsley
- 1 onion, sliced
- 2 tablespoons capers
- Salt and pepper, to taste

How To

1. Take a heavy-bottomed pot and place it over high heat for 2 minutes.
2. Add oil, heat it up for 2 minutes.
3. Stir in onion and garlic.
4. Sauté for 5 minutes.
5. Add remaining ingredients except for parsley.
6. Stir fry for 10 minutes.

7. Season accordingly and serve with a sprinkle of parsley.
8. Enjoy!

Nutrition Values (Per Serving)

- Calories: 331
- Fat: 4g
- Carbohydrates: 2g
- Protein: 22g

Perfect Caesar Salad

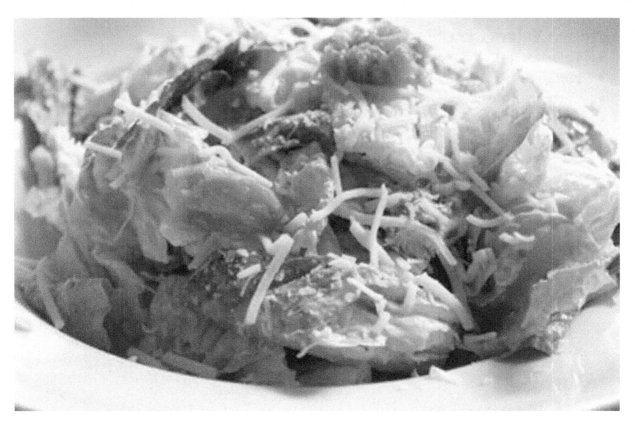

Serving: 2

Prep Time: 10 minutes

Cook Time: 0 minute

Ingredients

- 6 tablespoons cashew cheese
- ½ cup low-fat mayonnaise
- 1 teaspoon Worcestershire sauce
- 1 tablespoon lemon juice
- 1 teaspoon Dijon mustard
- 1 head romaine lettuce, torn into bite-sized
- 5 anchovy filets, minced
- 1 tablespoon lemon juice
- Ground pepper, to taste
- Salt, to taste

How To

1. Take a small bowl and add lemon juice, mustard, Worcestershire sauce, 1/3 of parmesan cheese, mayonnaise, anchovies, and garlic.

2. Whisk them well and season with salt and pepper.
3. Set aside in the refrigerator.
4. Take another bowl and place lettuce and pour in the dressing.
5. Toss well to coat.
6. Add remaining parmesan cheese on top.
7. Serve and enjoy!

Nutrition Values (Per Serving)

- Calories: 199
- Fat: 9g
- Carbohydrates: 15g
- Protein: 10g

Epic Glazed Salmon

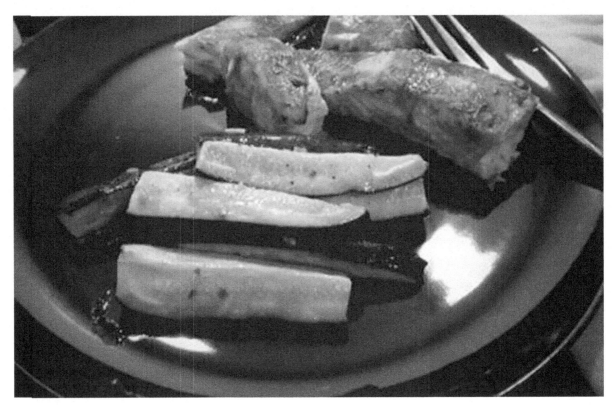

Serving: 4

Prep Time: 45 minutes

Cook Time: 10 minutes

Ingredients

- 4 pieces salmon fillets, 5 ounces each
- 4 tablespoons coconut aminos
- 4 teaspoon olive oil
- 2 teaspoon ginger, minced
- 4 teaspoon garlic, minced
- 2 tablespoon sugar-free ketchup
- 4 tablespoons dry white wine
- 2 tablespoons red boat fish sauce

How To

1. Take a bowl and mix in coconut aminos, garlic, ginger, fish sauce, and mix.

2. Add salmon and let it marinate for 15-20 minutes.

3. Take a skillet/pan and place it over medium heat.

4. Add oil and let it heat up.

5. Add salmon fillets and cook on HIGH for 3-4 minutes per side.

6. Remove dish once crispy.

7. Add sauce and wine.

8. Simmer for 5 minutes on low heat.

9. Return salmon to the glaze and flip until both sides are glazed.

10. Serve and enjoy!

Nutrition (Per Serving)

- Calories: 372
- Fat: 24g
- Carbohydrates: 3g
- Protein: 35g

Creamy Coconut Shrimp Curry

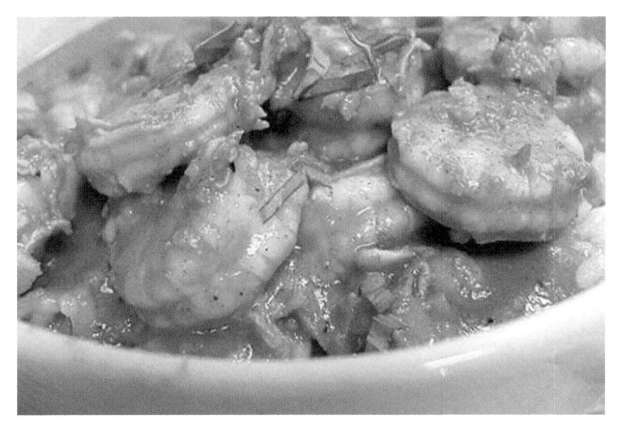

Serving: 4

Prep Time: 10 minutes

Cook Time: nil

Ingredients

- 1 pound shrimp, cooked, peeled, and deveined
- 1 tablespoon coconut cream
- ¼ teaspoon jalapeno, chopped
- ½ teaspoon lime juice
- 1 tablespoon parsley, chopped
- Pinch of pepper

How To

1. Take a bowl and add shrimp, cream, jalapeno, lime juice, parsley, pepper.
2. Toss well and divide into small bowls.
3. Serve and enjoy!

Nutrition Values (Per Serving)

- Calories: 183
- Fat: 5g
- Net Carbohydrates: 12g
- Protein: 8g

Prawn and Rice Croquettes

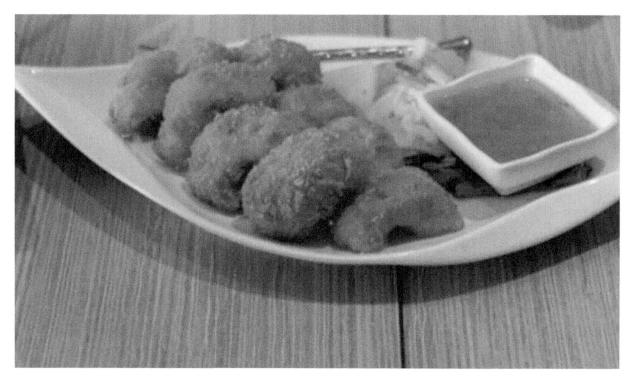

Serving: 8

Prep Time: 25 minute

Cook Time: 13 minutes

Ingredients

- 2 tablespoons almond butter
- ½ onion, chopped
- 4 ounces shrimp, peeled and chopped
- 2 tablespoons all-purpose flour
- 1 tablespoon white wine
- ½ cup almond milk
- 2 tablespoons almond milk
- 2 cups cooked rice
- 1 tablespoon parmesan, grated
- 1 teaspoon fresh dill, chopped
- 1 teaspoon sunflower seeds
- Ground pepper as needed
- Vegetable oil for frying
- 3 tablespoons all-purpose flour
- 1 whole egg

- ½ cup breadcrumbs

How To

1. Take a large skillet and place it over medium heat; add almond butter and let it melt.

2. Add onion, cook, and stir for 5 minutes.

3. Add shrimp and cook for 1-2 minutes.

4. Stir in 2 tablespoons flour, white wine, pour in almond milk gradually, and cook for 3-5 minutes until the sauce thickens.

5. Remove white sauce from heat and stir in rice, mix evenly.

6. Add dill, sunflower seeds, pepper and let it cool for 15 minutes.

7. Heat oil in a large saucepan and bring it to 350 degrees F.

8. Take a bowl and whisk in the egg, spread breadcrumbs on a plate.

9. Form rice mixture into 8 balls and roll 1 ball in flour, dip in egg and coat with crumbs, repeat with all balls.

10. Deep fry balls for 3 minutes.

11. Enjoy!

Nutrition Values (Per Serving)

- Calories: 182
- Fat: 7g
- Carbohydrates: 21g
- Protein: 7g

Sesame and Miso Salmon

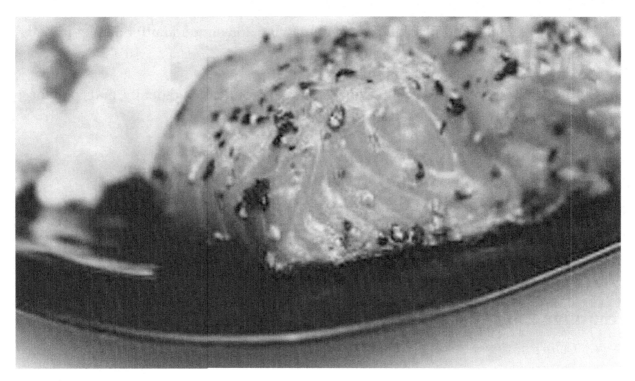

Serving: 6

Prep Time: 5 minutes

Cook Time: 10 minutes

Ingredients

- 2 ½ pound salmon fillets, skin removed
- 1 thumb-sized ginger, grated
- 2 tablespoons sesame seeds
- 1 teaspoon sesame oil
- ¼ cup of water
- 1 cup miso paste
- 3 tablespoons of rice wine vinegar

How To

1. Take a heavy-bottomed pot on medium-high heat.
2. Heat the pot for 2 minutes.
3. Add all ingredients and mix them well.
4. Cover it and bring to a boil.
5. Boil for 2 minutes and lower the heat.
6. Simmer for 10 minutes.
7. Serve and enjoy!

Nutrition Values (Per Serving)

- Calories: 343
- Fat: 12g
- Carbohydrates: 12g
- Protein: 44g

Perfectly Broiled Lamb Chops

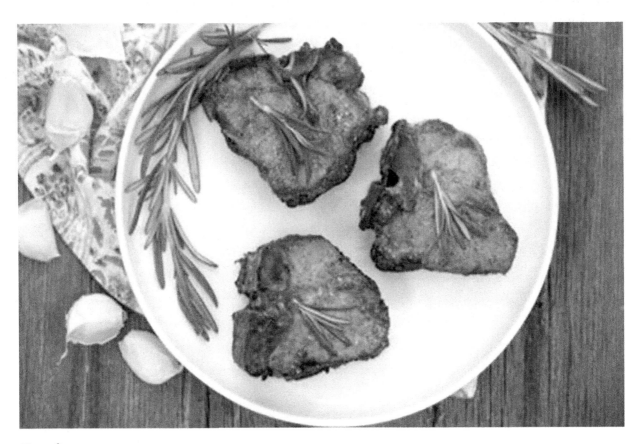

Serving: 4

Prep Time: 10 minutes

Cook Time: 10 minutes

Ingredients

- 8 pieces(4 ounces each) lamb loin chops
- 1 tablespoon bottled garlic, minced
- 2 tablespoons lemon juice
- ½ teaspoon salt
- ¼ teaspoon black pepper
- 1 tablespoon oregano, dried
- Cooking spray

How To

1. Preheat your broiler.
2. Take a big bowl, combine black pepper, garlic, lemon juice, salt, and oregano
3. Rub on all sides of lamb chops equally.
4. Coat a broiler pan with cooking spray before placing the lamb chops on the pan.

5. Broil 5 minutes for each side.
6. Serve and enjoy!

Nutrition Values (Per Serving)

- Calories: 332
- Fat: 16g
- Carbohydrates: 3g
- Protein: 46g

Traditional Black Bean Chili

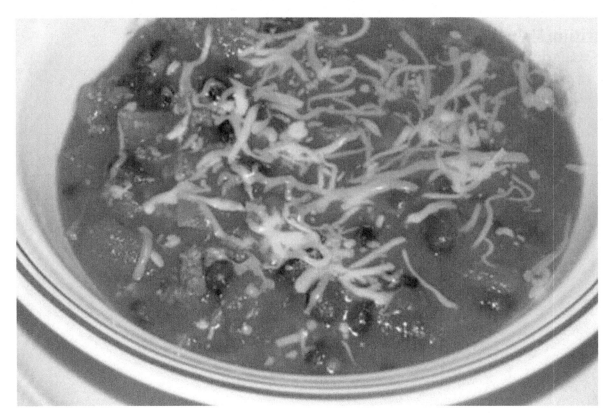

Serving: 4

Prep Time: 10 minutes

Cooking Time: 4 hours

Ingredients:

- 1 ½ cups red bell pepper, chopped
- 1 cup yellow onion, chopped
- 1 ½ cups mushrooms, sliced
- 1 tablespoon olive oil
- 1 tablespoon chili powder
- 2 garlic cloves, minced
- 1 teaspoon chipotle chili pepper, chopped
- ½ teaspoon cumin, ground
- 16 ounces canned black beans, drained and rinsed
- 2 tablespoons cilantro, chopped
- 1 cup tomatoes, chopped

How To:

1. Add red bell peppers, onion, dill, mushrooms, chili powder, garlic, chili pepper, cumin, black beans, tomatoes to your Slow Cooker.
2. Stir well.
3. Place lid and cook on HIGH for 4 hours.
4. Sprinkle cilantro on top.
5. Serve and enjoy!

Nutritional Contents:

- Calories: 211
- Fat: 3g
- Carbohydrates: 22g
- Protein: 5g

Healthy Tuna Croquettes

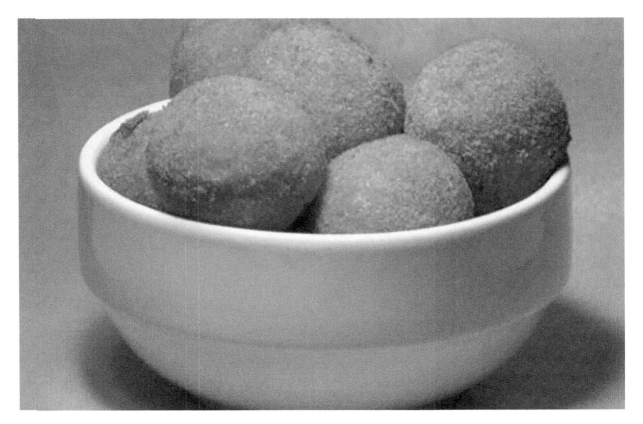

Serving: 4

Prep Time: 4 minutes

Cook Time: 9 minutes

Ingredients

- 1 can tuna, drained
- 1 whole large egg
- 8 tablespoons cashew cheese
- 2 tablespoons flax meal
- Salt and pepper to taste
- 1 tablespoon onion, minced

How To

1. Add all of the ingredients to a blender (except flax meal) and pulse the mixture into a crunchy texture.
2. Form patties using the mixture.
3. Dip both sides of the patties in flax meal and fry them in hot oil until both sides are browned well.

Nutrition (Per Serving)

- Calories: 105
- Fat: 5g
- Carbohydrates: 2g
- Protein: 14g

Juicy Steamed Garlic Halibut

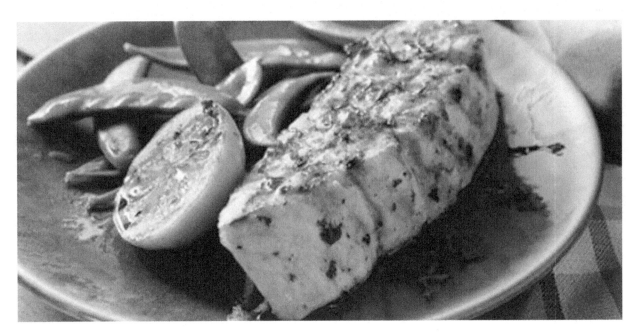

Serving: 4

Prep Time: 5 minutes

Cook Time: 25 minutes

Ingredients

- 1 pound halibut fillet
- 1 lemon, freshly squeezed
- 1 tablespoon dill weed, chopped
- 1 teaspoon garlic powder
- Salt and pepper to taste

How To

1. Take a large pot and fill up with 1.5 inches of water.
2. Place it over medium heat.
3. Place a trivet inside the pot.
4. Take a baking dish small enough to fit inside the pot.
5. Add listed ingredients and gently stir.
6. Cover the baking dish with foil.
7. Place it over the top on the trivet inside the pot.
8. Cover the pot and steam fish for 15 minutes.
9. Keep the fish for 10 minutes before removing it from the pot.
10. Serve and enjoy!

Nutrition Values (Per Serving)

- Calories: 270
- Fat: 6.5g
- Carbohydrates: 1.8g
- Protein: 47.8g

Sun-Dried Tomatoes and Salmon

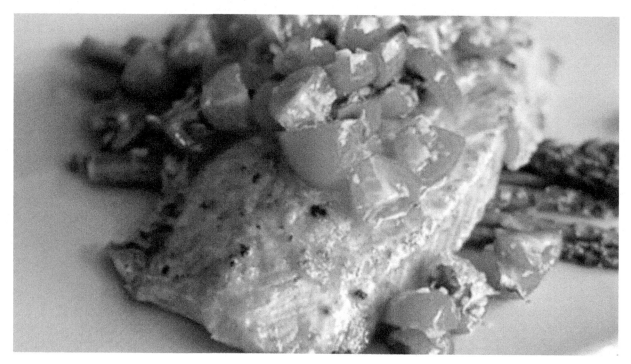

Serving: 2

Prep Time: 10 minutes

Cook Time: 15 minutes

Ingredients

- 1 salmon fillet
- 2 tablespoons sun-dried tomatoes, chopped
- ¼ teaspoon cayenne pepper
- 1 tablespoon capers
- ½ teaspoon thyme, dried
- ½ lemon, freshly squeezed
- ½ teaspoon oregano, dried
- 2 cloves garlic, minced
- ¼ cup of water
- Salt and pepper, to taste

How To

1. Take a heavy-bottomed pot over medium-high heat.
2. Add all ingredients.
3. Mix well, then cover to bring the boil.
4. Once boiling, reduce the heat and let simmer for 10 minutes.

5. Adjust seasoning to taste and cook for 3 minutes.

6. Serve and enjoy!

Nutrition Values (Per Serving)

- Calories: 265
- Fat: 8g
- Carbohydrates: 6g
- Protein: 10g

Almond and Butter Shrimp

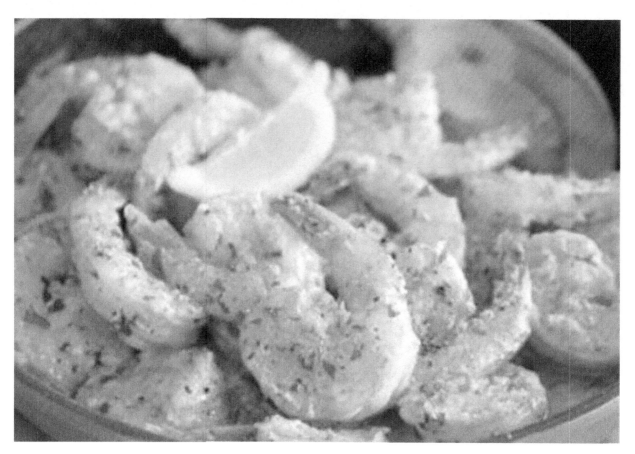

Serving: 4

Prep Time: 15 minutes

Cook Time: 30 minutes

Ingredients

- 4 pounds shrimp
- 1-2 tablespoons garlic, minced
- ½ cup almond butter
- 1 tablespoon lemon pepper seasoning
- ½ teaspoon garlic powder

How To

1. Preheat your oven to 300 degrees F.
2. Take a bowl and mix in garlic and almond butter.
3. Place shrimp in a pan and dot with almond butter garlic mix.
4. Sprinkle garlic powder and lemon pepper.
5. Bake for 30 minutes.

6. Enjoy!

Nutrition Values (Per Serving)

- Calories: 749
- Fat: 30g
- Net Carbohydrates: 7g
- Protein: 74g

Extreme Balsamic Chicken

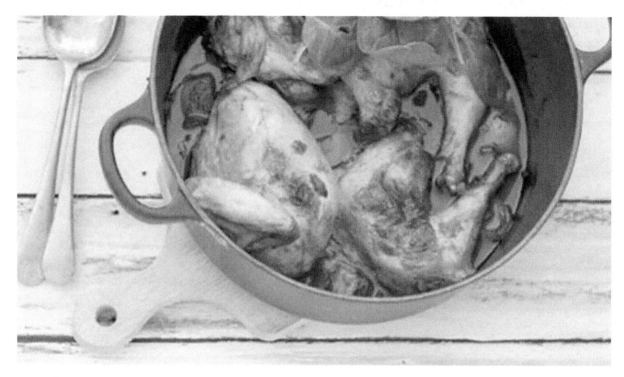

Serving: 4

Prep Time: 10 minutes

Cook Time: 35 minutes

Ingredients

- 3 boneless chicken breast, skinless
- Sunflower seeds to taste
- ¼ cup of almond flour
- 2/3 cup of low-fat chicken broth
- 1 ½ teaspoons of arrowroot
- ½ cup of low sugar raspberry preserve
- 1 ½ tablespoons of balsamic vinegar

How To

1. Cut chicken breast into bite-sized pieces and season them with seeds.

2. Dredge the chicken pieces in flour and shake off any excess.

3. Take a non-stick skillet and place it over medium heat.

4. Add chicken to the skillet and cook for 15 minutes, making sure to turn them halfway through.

5. Remove chicken and transfer to a platter.

6. Add arrowroot, broth, raspberry preserve to the skillet and stir.

7. Stir in balsamic vinegar and reduce heat to low, stir cook for a few minutes.

8. Transfer the chicken back to the sauce and cook for 15 minutes more.

9. Serve and enjoy!

<u>Nutrition Values (Per Serving)</u>

- Calories: 546
- Fat: 35g
- Carbohydrates: 11g
- Protein: 44g

Chapter 8: Bonus Smoothies
Cool Strawberry Shake

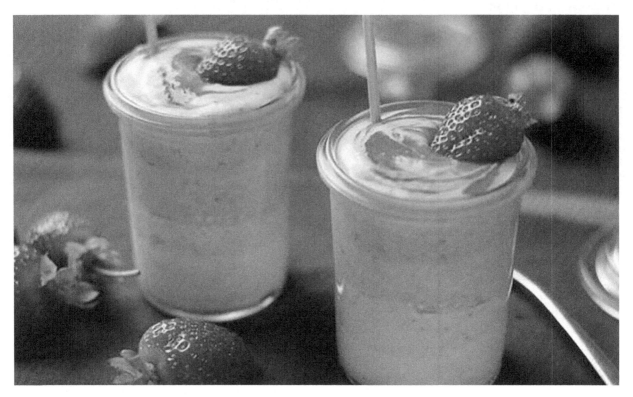

Serving: 1

Prep Time: 10 minutes

Ingredients:

- ½ cup cashew cream, liquid
- 1 tablespoon cocoa powder
- 1 pack stevia
- ½ cup strawberry, sliced
- 1 tablespoon coconut flakes, unsweetened
- 1 ½ cups of water

How To:

1. Add listed ingredients to a blender.
2. Blend until you have a smooth and creamy texture.
3. Serve chilled and enjoy!

Nutritional Contents:

- Calories: 470

- Fat: 46g
- Carbohydrates: 15g
- Protein: 4g

Generous Coffee Smoothie

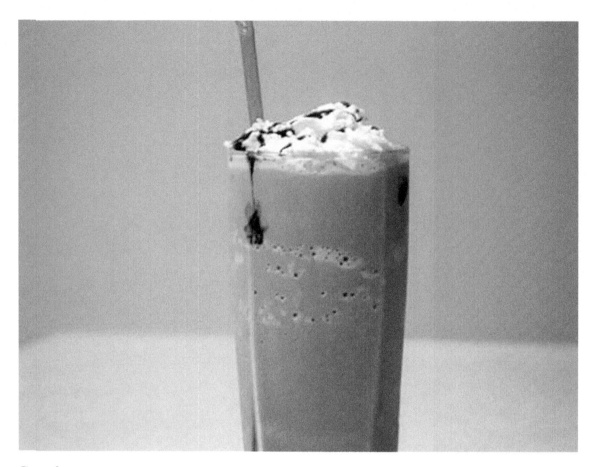

Serving: 1

Prep Time: 10 minutes

Ingredients:

- 1 tablespoon chia seeds
- 2 cups strongly brewed coffee, chilled
- 1-ounce Macadamia Nuts
- 1-2 packets Stevia, optional
- 1 tablespoon MCT oil

How To:

1. Add all the listed ingredients to a blender.
2. Blend on high until smooth and creamy.
3. Enjoy your smoothie.

Nutritional Contents:

- Calories: 395
- Fat: 39g

- Carbohydrates: 11g
- Protein: 5.2g

Apple and Berry Packed Smoothie

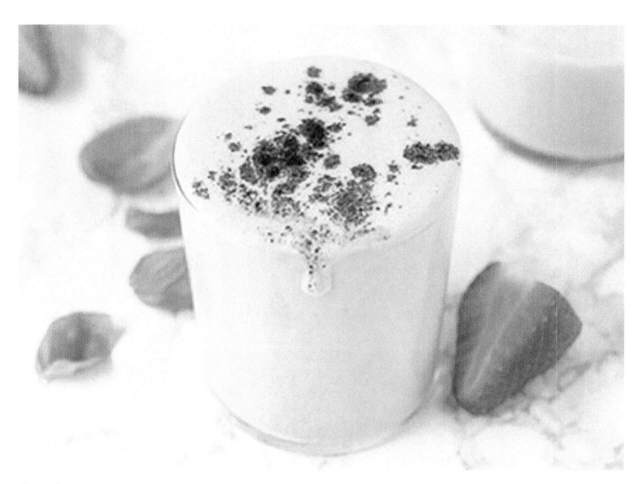

Serving: 2

Prep Time: 5 minutes

Ingredients

- 2 cups frozen blackberries
- ½ cup apple cider
- 1 apple, cubed
- 2/3 cup non-fat lemon yogurt

How To

1. Add the listed ingredients to your blender and blend until smooth.
2. Serve chilled!

Nutrition (Per Serving)

- Calories: 200
- Fat: 10g

- Carbohydrates: 14g
- Protein 2g

Berrylicious Green Smoothie

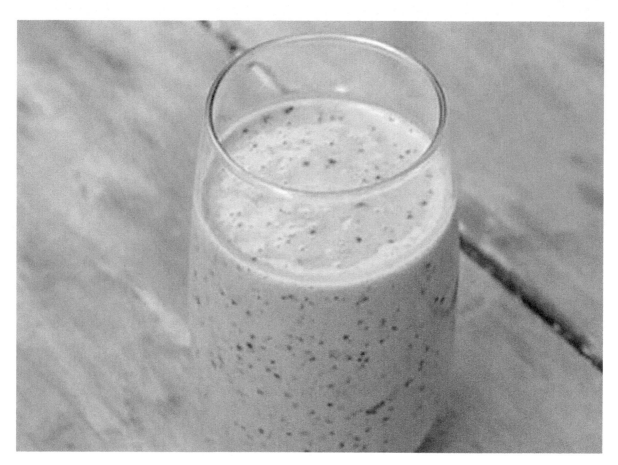

Serving: 2

Prep Time: 5 minutes

Ingredients

- 1 cup spinach leaves
- ½ cup frozen blueberries
- 1 ripe banana
- ½ cup almond milk
- 2 tablespoons old fashioned oats
- ½ tablespoon stevia

Cooking How-To

1. Add the listed ingredients to your blender and blend until smooth.
2. Serve chilled!

Nutrition (Per Serving)

- Calories: 200

- Fat: 10g
- Carbohydrates: 14g
- Protein 2g

Ginger and Berry Smoothie

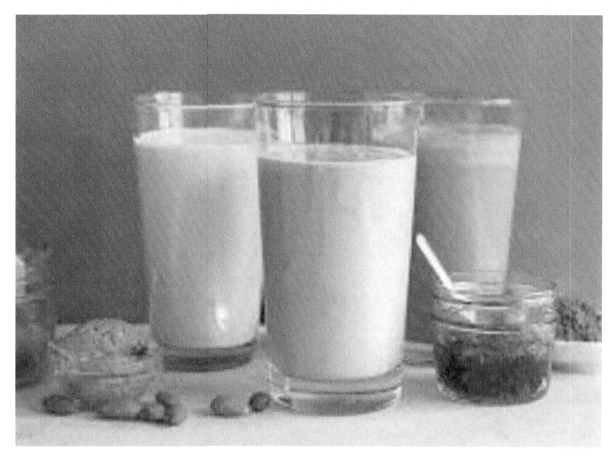

Serving: 2

Prep Time: 5 minutes

Cook Time: Nil

Ingredients

- 2 cups blackberries
- 2 cups unsweetened almond milk
- 1 -2 packs of stevia
- 1 piece of 1-inch fresh ginger, peeled and roughly chopped
- 2 cups crushed ice

How To

1. Add the listed ingredients to a blender and blend the whole mixture until smooth.
2. Serve chilled and enjoy!

Nutrition (Per Serving)

- Calories: 200
- Fat: 10g
- Carbohydrates: 14g
- Protein 2g

Chilled Coconut and Hazelnut Glass

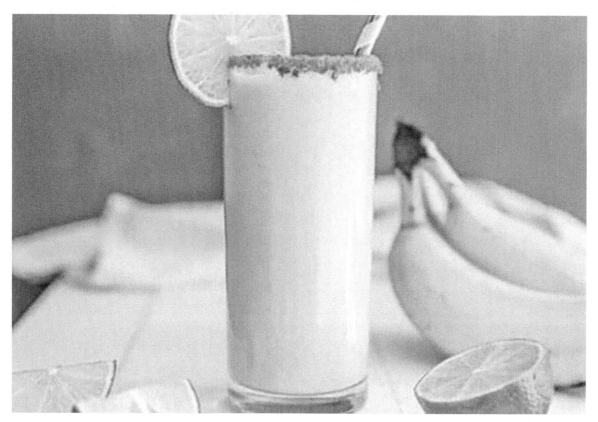

Serving: 1

Prep Time: 10 minutes

Ingredients:

- ½ cup coconut almond milk
- ¼ cup hazelnuts, chopped
- 1 ½ cups of water
- 1 pack stevia

How To:

1. Add listed ingredients to a blender.

2. Blend until you have a smooth and creamy texture.

3. Serve chilled and enjoy!

Nutritional Values (Per Serving)

- Calories: 457
- Fat: 46g
- Carbohydrates: 12g
- Protein: 7g

Original Mocha Shake

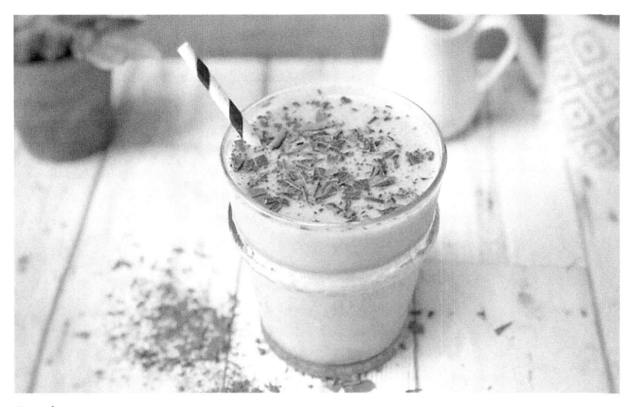

Serving: 1

Prep Time: 10 minutes

Ingredients:

- 1 cup whole almond milk
- 2 tablespoons cocoa powder
- 2 pack stevia
- 1 cup brewed coffee, chilled
- 1 tablespoon coconut oil

How To:

1. Add listed ingredients to a blender.

2. Blend until you have a smooth and creamy texture.

3. Serve chilled and enjoy!

Nutritional Contents:

- Calories: 293
- Fat: 23g
- Carbohydrates: 19g
- Protein: 10g

Cinnamon Chiller

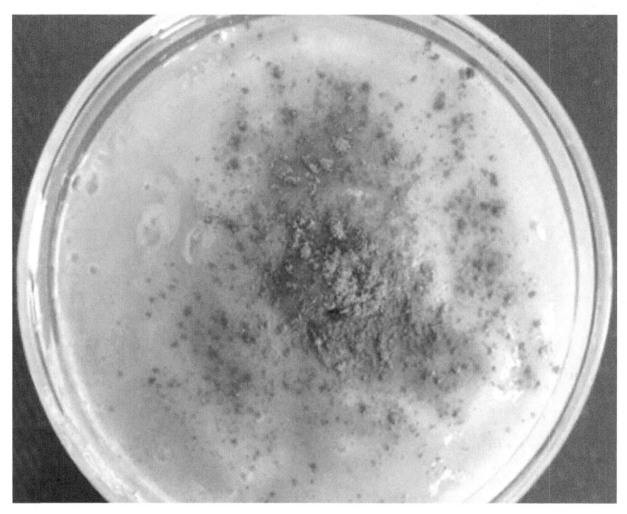

Serving: 1

Prep Time: 10 minutes

Ingredients:

- 1 cup unsweetened almond milk
- 2 tablespoons vanilla protein powder
- ½ teaspoon cinnamon
- ¼ teaspoon vanilla extract
- 1 tablespoon chia seeds
- 1 cup ice cubes

How To:

1. Add listed ingredients to a blender.

2. Blend until you have a smooth and creamy texture.

3. Serve chilled and enjoy!

Nutritional Contents:

- Calories: 145
- Fat: 4g
- Carbohydrates: 1.6g
- Protein: 0.6g

Strawberry Alkaline Smoothie

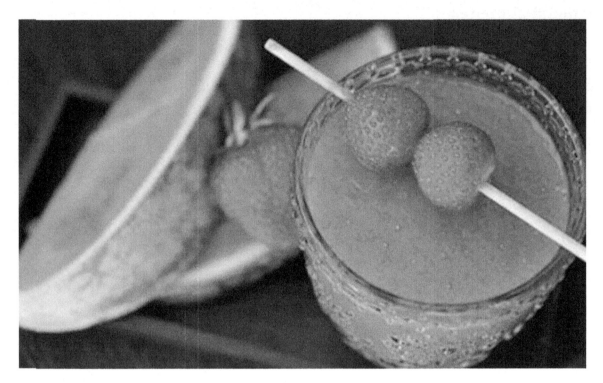

Serving: 2

Prep Time: 5 minutes

Ingredients

- ½ cup of organic strawberries/blueberries
- Half a banana
- 2 cups of coconut water
- ½ inch ginger
- Juice of 2 grapefruits

How To

1. Add all the listed ingredients to your blender.
2. Blend until smooth.
3. Add a few ice cubes and serve the smoothie.
4. Enjoy!

Nutrition (Per Serving)

- Calories: 200
- Fat: 10g
- Carbohydrates: 14g
- Protein 2g

Pineapple and Coconut Milky Smoothie

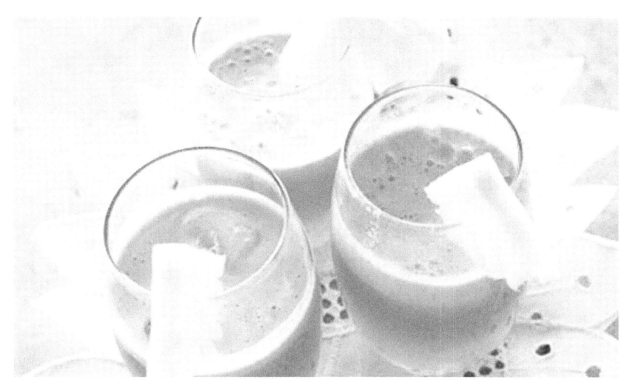

Serving: 2

Prep Time: 5 minutes

Ingredients

- ¼ cup pineapple, frozen
- ¾ cup of coconut milk

How To

1. Add the listed ingredients to a blender and blend well on high.

2. Once the mixture is smooth, pour the smoothie into a tall glass and serve.

3. Chill and enjoy it!

Nutrition (Per Serving)

- Calories: 200
- Fat: 10g
- Carbohydrates: 14g
- Protein 2g

Pineapple and Apple Smoothie

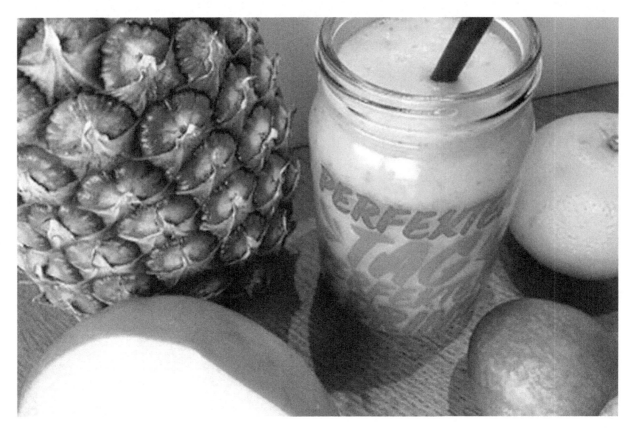

Serving: 1

Prep Time: 10 minutes

Cook Time: 0 minute

Ingredients

- 2 cups pineapple, cubed
- 2 apples, cored
- 8 ounces almond milk
- 1 head escarole lettuce
- 1 stalk celery

How To

1. Add all ingredients to your blender.
2. Blend it until you get a smooth and creamy mixture.
3. Serve chilled and enjoy!

Nutrition Values (Per Serving)
- Calories: 466

- Fat: 8g
- Carbohydrates: 103g
- Protein: 8g

Anti-Inflam Blueberry Glass

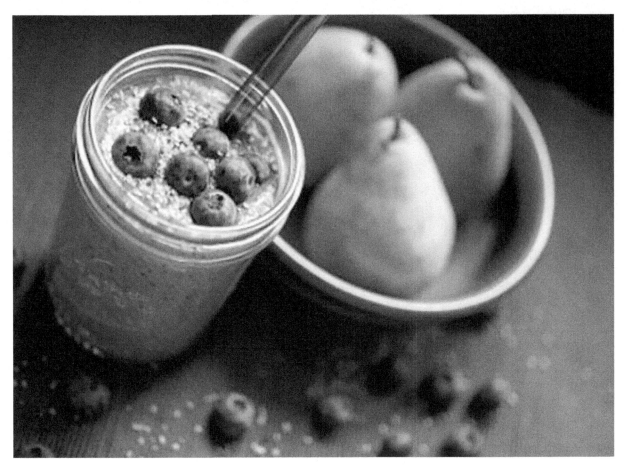

Serving: 1

Prep Time: 5 minutes

Cook Time: 0 minutes

Ingredients

- 1 cup blueberries, frozen
- 1 cup almond milk
- 1 tablespoon almond butter
- 2 handfuls spinach
- ¼ teaspoon cinnamon
- 1 teaspoon maca powder
- ¼ teaspoon cayenne pepper

How To

1. Add all the ingredients to a blender.
2. Blend until mix well.

3. Serve immediately and enjoy!

Nutrition Values (Per Serving)

- Calories: 431
- Fat: 4g
- Carbohydrates: 56g
- Protein: 10g

Healthy Trio-Smoothie

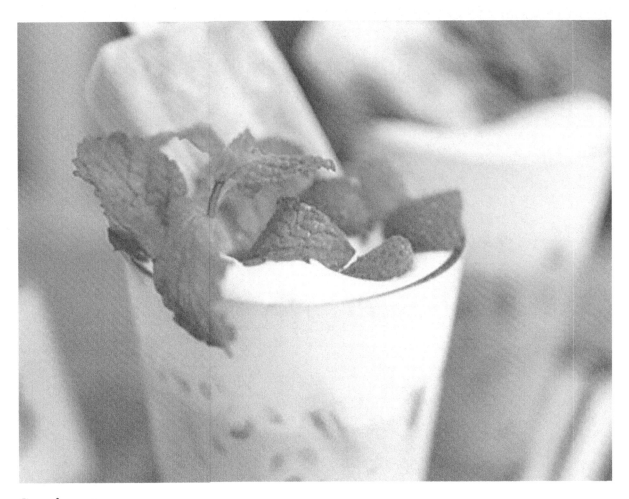

Serving: 1

Prep Time: 10 minutes

Cook Time: 0 minute

Ingredients

- ¼ cup 100% whole grain oats, rolled
- ½ cup Greek yogurt, plain
- ¼ cup kale, shredded and stems discarded
- ½ cup of ice
- 2 teaspoons flaxseed
- ½ banana, peeled
- 1 teaspoon honey
- ½ cup almond milk

How To

1. Add all ingredients to your blender.
2. Blend it until you get a smooth and creamy mixture.
3. Serve chilled and enjoy!

Nutrition Values (Per Serving)

- Calories: 305
- Fat: 10g
- Carbohydrates: 54g
- Protein: 11g

Tart Cherry and Greens Smoothie

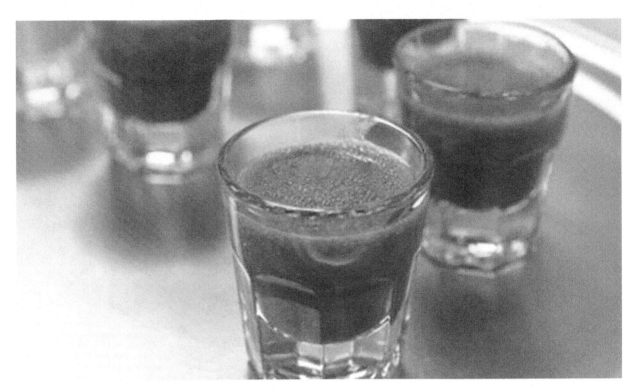

Serving: 1

Prep Time: 10 minutes

Cook Time: 0 minute

Ingredients

- 1 cup tart cherry, frozen and pitted
- 1/2 cup kale, stems removed and chopped
- 1/2 cup broccoli florets
- 1/2 cup orange juice, squeezed
- 1/2 cup cold water

How To

1. Add puree cherries, kale, orange juice, broccoli to your blender.
2. Blend it until smooth and creamy.
3. Add remaining ingredients and blend it until you get a smooth mixture.
4. Serve and enjoy!

Nutrition Values (Per Serving)

- Calories: 157
- Fat: 0.6g

- Carbohydrates: 37g
- Protein: 4g

Green Tea and Raspberry Chiller

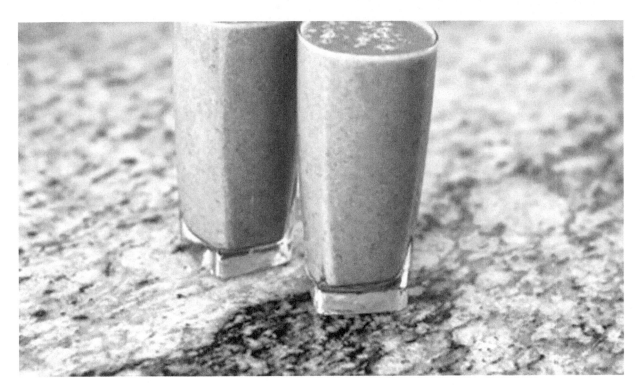

Serving: 2

Prep Time: 10 minutes

Cook Time: 0 minute

Ingredients

- 1 banana
- 1 tablespoon honey
- 2 cups raspberries, frozen and unsweetened
- 1/4 cup protein powder
- 1 1/2 cups chilled green tea

How To

1. Add all ingredients to your blender.
2. Blend it until you get a smooth mixture.
3. Serve and enjoy!

Nutrition Values (Per Serving)

- Calories: 241
- Fat: 5g
- Carbohydrates: 41g

- Protein: 12.5g

The Super Green Detox

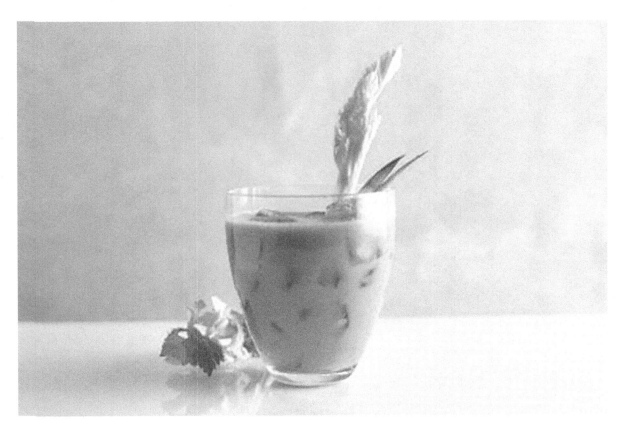

Serving: 2

Prep Time: 10 minutes

Cook Time: 0 minute

Ingredients

- 1 cup orange or tangerine juice, chilled
- 2 medium ribs celery, chopped
- 1/4 cup mint leaves, chopped
- 1/4 cup leaf parsley, chopped
- 1 1/4 cups mango, frozen cubes
- 1 1/4 cups kale, stems and ribs removed
- 1 cucumber, peeled
- 2-3 dates, for sweetness, optional
- 6 ice cubes

How To

1. Add all ingredients to your blender.
2. Blend it until you get a smooth mixture.
3. Serve and enjoy!

Nutrition Values (Per Serving)

- Calories: 160
- Fat: 0g
- Carbohydrates: 39g
- Protein: 3g

Beans, Peaches and Greens Smoothie

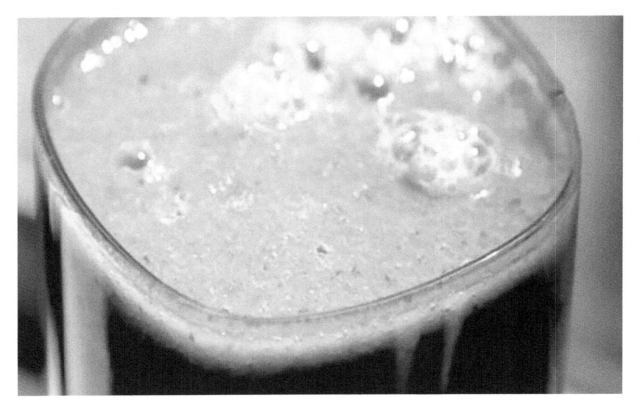

Serving: 1

Prep Time: 10 minutes

Cook Time: 0 minute

Ingredients

- 1 cup peaches, frozen
- 1/4 can white beans
- 1/2 cup almond milk
- 1/4 cup almond
- 1/4 cup quick-cooking oats
- 1/8 teaspoon cinnamon
- Pinch of nutmeg
- 1 cup packed lettuce
- 1/4 cup Italian parsley
- 6 ice cubes

How To

1. Add all ingredients to your blender.
2. Blend it until you get a smooth and creamy mixture.

3. Serve chilled and enjoy!

<u>Nutrition Values (Per Serving)</u>

- Calories: 346
- Fat: 11g
- Carbohydrates: 55g
- Protein: 12g

Cabbage and Coconut Chia Smoothie

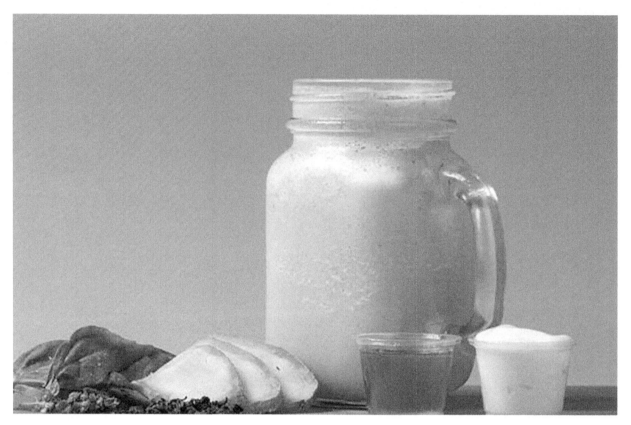

Serving: 2

Prep Time: 5 minutes

Ingredients

- 1/3 cup cabbage
- 1 cup cold unsweetened coconut milk
- 1 tablespoon chia seeds
- ½ cup cherries
- ½ cup spinach

How To

1. Add coconut milk to your blender.
2. Cut cabbage and add to your blender.
3. Place chia seeds in a coffee grinder and chop to powder; brush the powder into a blender.
4. Pit the cherries and add them to the blender.
5. Wash and dry the spinach and chop.
6. Add to the mix.
7. Cover and blend on low followed by medium.

8. Taste the texture and serve chilled!

<u>Nutrition (Per Serving)</u>

- Calories: 200
- Fat: 10g
- Carbohydrates: 14g
- Protein 2g

Ginger-Pear Smoothie

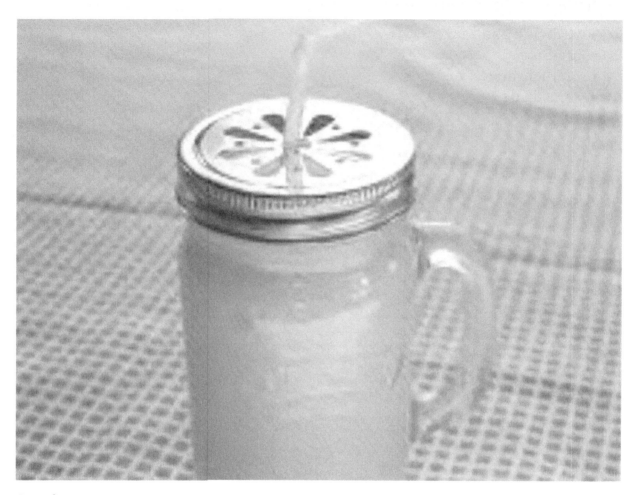

Serving: 1

Prep Time: 10 minutes

Cook Time: 0 minute

Ingredients

- 1 large ripe pear, cored and quartered
- 1 tablespoon ginger, peeled and chopped
- 1/4 cup whole almonds
- 2 cups baby spinach
- 1 tablespoon fresh lemon juice
- 3/4 cup cold water

How To

1. Add all ingredients to your blender.
2. Blend it until you get a smooth mixture.

3. Serve chilled and enjoy!

Nutrition Values (Per Serving)

- Calories: 154
- Fat: 8g
- Carbohydrates: 13g
- Protein: 8g

Cherry Almond Smoothie

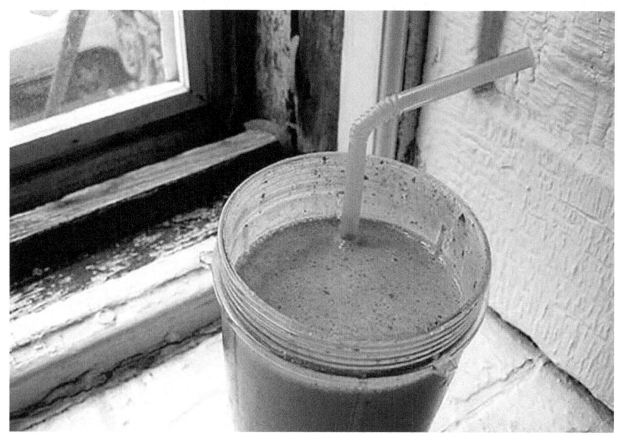

Serving: 4

Prep Time: 3 hours

Cook Time: 0 minute

Ingredients

- 2 cups sweet cherries, pitted
- ¾ cup chia seeds
- ¼ cup maple syrup
- ½ cup hemp seeds
- 2 cups of coconut milk
- 1 teaspoon vanilla extract
- 1/8 teaspoon salt

How To

1. Add cherries, coconut milk, salt, vanilla extract, and maple syrup into your blender.
2. Blend until smooth.
3. Divide chia seeds and hemp seeds into 4 glasses.

4. Pour in the cherry and milk mixture.

5. Let it chill for 3 hours.

6. Serve and enjoy!

<u>Nutrition Values (Per Serving)</u>

- Calories: 302
- Fat: 4g
- Carbohydrates: 29g
- Protein: 10g

Conclusion

I would like to thank you again for purchasing the book and taking the time to go through it.

I hope that this book has been helpful and you found the information useful!

Keep in mind that you are not only limited to the recipes provided in this book! Just keep on exploring until you find the best Anti-Inflammatory regime that works for you!

Stay healthy and stay safe!

Made in the USA
Middletown, DE
11 June 2021